SEP 2 2 1978

The Catholic
Theological Union
LIBRARY
Chicago, Ill.

MEDICINE, SCIENCE AND LIFE

MEDICINE, SCIENCE AND LIFE

by
V. S. Yanovsky

The Catholic
Theological Union
LIBRARY
Chicago, Ill.

WITHDRAWN

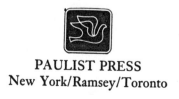

PAULIST PRESS
New York/Ramsey/Toronto

Copyright © 1978 by
V. S. Yanovsky

All rights reserved. No part of this book may be reproduced or transmitted in any form or by any means, electronic or mechanical, including photocopying, recording or by any information storage and retrieval system without permission in writing from the Publisher.

Library of Congress
Catalog Card Number: 77-99304

ISBN: 0-8091-2094-1

Published by Paulist Press
Editorial Office: 1865 Broadway, New York, N.Y. 10023
Business Office: 545 Island Road, Ramsey, N.J. 07446

Printed and bound in the
United States of America

CONTENTS

"And I vowed that, if God should ever give me the means, I would do something to redress the grievances and relieve the sufferings of that class of beings with whom my lot had so long been cast."

Two Years Before the Mast
Richard Henry Dana, Jr.

FOREWORD

On the eleventh floor of the big hospital are the operating rooms. At dawn the OR is a picture of ideal order, logic, technical progress. Shortly before eight o'clock the first patient is wheeled in and put to sleep. Half an hour later the same room seems completely transformed—the confusion, the smells, puddles, and discarded trash evoke a battlefield where soldiers, forgetting all they have been taught at games and drills, act according to the situation, just trying to do their best.

The new sophisticated suction machine has broken down and has to be hastily replaced by two obsolete ones; the ingenious reflector does not throw back light at the needed angle; a floor spotlight has been connected and the nurses get entangled in the extension cord; a pint of blood has fallen off the hook—the circulating nurse starts mopping up but the surgeon asks for a smaller drain and she disappears to fetch one; the obese assistant wants his forehead wiped continuously to prevent his sweat from dripping into the wound (it is much too hot but the central steam heat cannot be turned off).

I recall a particularly gloomy November morning. Life seemed suspended in the operating room. The surgeon resembled a boxer who, his right ready for the blow, has been stopped dead by the bell and has to preserve the punch for the next round. We were operating on a breast tumor, performing a frozen section. The mass is excised and sent to the lab where a microscopic analysis of the tumor is made by the pathologist within ten or fifteen minutes. Surgeon, assistants, nurses, anesthesiologist—perhaps even the woman asleep on the table—all were waiting tensely. Five minutes passed, and five more. "A good sign," the surgeon said; "they usually spot a malignant tumor right away." Presently the answer from the laboratory would come: simple adenoma! The surgeon would crack a joke and swiftly put in the stitches; with smiles of relief the others would begin to tidy up in anticipation of the next case.

Half an hour later the patient would be on the ward, discharged from the hospital in two or three days, and the incident seemingly closed.

But another answer is also possible: atypical mytosis of the cells—cancer! Then the long, difficult, painful process of a radical operation would begin. The patient would be in bed for weeks, receive postoperative X-ray treatment and chemotherapy, and for years be under medical supervision (with the outcome doubtful). Such is the difference—life and death are concentrated in that span of a quarter of an hour while we wait for the answer from the laboratory.

Almost twenty minutes had passed. Everybody was getting very tense. In this particular case (perhaps because the patient happened to be young and attractive?) I found the trial inordinately hard to endure. The surgeon was pacing up and down, keeping his bloodstained, gloved hands close to the chest in order not to contaminate them. Then, although we had all been expecting it, the answer came quite unexpectedly. "Benign cyst!" As I once more automatically looked at the clock, a simple thought, sharp as a blade, struck me: What does the woman's husband feel at this moment? (I had caught a glimpse of him and the children before the operation.) How can they bear it?

And suddenly I saw us all as on a vast stage, participants in a drama that is being enacted in perpetuity.

There is the husband waiting for the verdict. He has, for better or worse, delivered his wife into the surgeon's hands, believing that the physician will be master of the situation. Here is the surgeon, sheepishly waiting for the answer from the lab (meanwhile protecting his disposable gloves). There is the pathologist staring into the microscope. Under the lens he does not find a label with an inscription—cyst, adenoma, cancer. He sees only an agglomeration of cells that he has to interpret, and this interpretation is difficult, full of pitfalls, and sometimes impossible to achieve. And here, presumably in good hands, is the patient, exposed and disarmed, who never quite realized the scope of the drama into which she stepped, unprepared, as the central character. On that November morning the idea for my book was born.

There is hardly a situation in life that equals in significance the appearance of the doctor at the sickbed. In the great crisis of illness and death the figure of the doctor is always present, reflecting our hopes and fears. During such decisive moments he seems to grow over-life size, superhuman, of more importance than the heroes and tyrants in a classic tragedy. This is how the patient sees him, wants to see him. Thus, even the worthiest of doctors, knowingly or unknowingly, is forced into a false position and gradually accepts it. He puts on a mask and plays the role that convention, society, and professional tradition have assigned to him.

What hides behind the facade, to what extent should we trust the physician and all other specialists—scientists armed with numerous credentials? What, as a matter of fact, is a scientist? How "scientific" are our sciences, how revealing and precise can they possibly be? Could it be that, instead of the so-called backward theological concepts and metaphysical speculations, we have created a new form of religion or, rather, a pseudo-religion where, instead of God, science is glorified, and, in place of the priest, the M.D. or Ph.D. celebrates the mass?

On that dreary morning, waiting for the results of the *frozen section*, conscientiously assisting the young woman in her labored breathing and thinking of her husband and children gathered downstairs, I promised myself—and all the unfortunates whose bodily integrity I had helped to assault for so many years—to try and answer those questions and thus contribute to an enlightened understanding of medicine and science in our life. I felt I owed it to all past and future patients, whose names are legion.

But that was easier to promise than to do. Very soon I found out that in order to develop a modern philosophy of medicine it was necessary, first of all, to establish a clear philosophy of life as a whole, since medicine by its very nature is interwoven with all aspects of our existence, physical as well as spiritual. In the last analysis, to answer the questions, "What is medicine? what can the physician's role in our life be (and what can it *not* be)?" we must first in all earnest define what *we* really are and what *we* were meant to be.

Religion speaks of eternal life and resurrection. Science seeks reversibility, in different forms according to its different branches: in medicine and biology it is the quest for well-being, rejuvenation, the return to a previous happy state of health and youth; in physics it is the partial or total overcoming of entropy (disorder). Art, with its fixation forever of objects or subjects in certain great or beautiful moments in time, fights against decay. All these projections of our existence must be understood and harmonized. Such is the scope and origin of my book.

In the first chapters I analyze three fields of medicine: anesthesia, surgery, and general medicine; how they work in our time and what their shortcomings are. These specialities were not chosen at random.

Anesthesia is a new discipline, supposedly the most pioneering, combining all fields of medicine, chemistry, and biophysics. It is also, by its very nature, reversibility par excellence. And reversibility is essential to medicine and to science in general.

Surgery is the most fashionable representative of modern medicine: heroic, aggressive, daring. Being essentially irreversible it is also, philosophically speaking, the antagonist of anesthesia.

General medicine is the basis of our profession—or should be. It is directed toward reversibility but, in its failures, often forgets this prime goal.

The last two parts of the book consist of a review of the old "modern" theories on which medicine was, *and still is*, based: gravitation, thermodynamics, classical evolution. The new quantum physics has made these theories obsolete—at least on the atomic and cellular level. But the changes in contemporary physics have not yet found an adequate expression in modern medicine.

It seems feasible and timely to project the essential concepts of the new quantum mechanics into our social and medical sciences (and also into art and religion). The fact is that Heisenberg's uncertainty principle applies to medicine and art as much as to physics. It means freedom of choice. Freedom of choice not only for every photon but for every cell and every person. Only in the framework of such freedom can a person grow, live and create, and eventually deal with physiological and pathological challenges.

Science, art, and religion must be brought together as one

team in the pursuit of the supreme reality, and this "unified field theory" became my basic aim.

Such an undertaking will probably antagonize some representatives of the disciplines studied here. As a matter of fact, this consideration kept me for a while from publishing this work. But finally I overcame my fear.

In his first year of philosophy and logic, the young student usually has to listen to the story of the ancient Greek who wanted to take up politics as a career. "My son," his mother told him, "don't do it. If you tell the truth the people will hate you, and if you tell lies the gods will hate you. In any event, some will hate you. Please do not go into politics!" The young man went away, saddened. But after a few days he returned joyously and declared: "Mother, I thought it over and I have decided to go into politics. If I tell the truth the gods will like me, and if I lie the people will like me. In any event, some will like me. I'll do it, mother dear!"

The author went through a somewhat similar experience.

Part I
ANESTHESIA

Anesthesia paralyzes the self-defense mechanism

I

Anesthesia may be characterized by the fact that a variety of medical problems requiring *immediate solution* meet very dramatically at the anesthesiologist's end of the table. Multiple disciplines—general physiology, cardiology, neurology, biochemistry, etc., etc.—converge suddenly, occupying, as it were, the same space at the same time. This *simultaneity* constitutes a definite, specific trait of anesthesia, its distinctive stamp. How to deal with it is not only a technical challenge, a demand upon scientific knowledge, but a philosophical problem as well: Time acquires a new meaning that must be explored.

Another inherent trait of anesthesia that also, and in an even more pointed way, brings up the problem of time is its *reversibility*. The abolished vital reflexes have to return; all complications, such as apnea, tachycardia, bradycardia, anoxia, are expected to disappear without leaving any traces. This means that reversibility is *conditio sine qua non*. But what is reversibility, philosophically speaking, if not a negation of time? "What has happened—can it unhappen?" as Kierkegaard has it. Generalized and applied to the whole of human life, reversibility can mean only one thing: the complete overcoming and negation of time and history.

Whatever its ultimate aim and reason, administration of anesthesia means intoxicating the patient. In fact, anesthesia is always evil, and the art is to choose between lesser and greater evil, not between good and evil. This is a trait anesthesia shares with the most crucial problems of contemporary life.

What first strikes the student of anesthesia and is, later, too easily forgotten or taken for granted is the anesthetist's unmitigated loneliness. We may, of course, consider that the people in the operating room are working on the patient as a team. However, this must be further elaborated. The surgeon has an assistant, even two or three if need be; the scrub nurse has a second scrub nurse, and a circulating nurse, and a bell to ring for more help; they are all working in the same operative field and in apparent communion! Only the anesthesiologist is on his own. The surgeon may ask him whether everything is going well, the kind circulating nurse may fetch him a larger airway, but those are minor, external contacts. Intellectually and spiritually the anesthesiologist is alone—facing that lesser evil.

The pathologist is in the lab with the specimen. He prepares the slides in a friendly atmosphere, can consult a book, make a telephone call to a colleague, and give an answer such as "frozen section not clear," "suspicious" (whatever that means), or "we need a paraffin preparation"; he can even send the slide by special delivery to Illinois or Massachusetts, correspond, deliberate, and then come up with the answer: "I don't know what it is—I once had a similar case—the patient died—apparently from a lymphosarcoma. . . ."

For obvious reasons, the anesthetist cannot do his work in such a fashion. He must always deliver the goods—here and now, by himself, in the presence of the impatient, often hostile, surgeon, and regardless of whether it "looks suspicious" or not, whether he has already had such a case or not.

In teaching institutions there might be, somewhere in an office or a hall, another anesthesiologist whom he could consult. But even here after 5 P.M. he is alone. Indeed, considering that the time element does not exist for him in the usual sense, the anesthetist really cannot be assisted from without, least of all in so-called private—i.e., commercial—institutions, where there are only competitors around. It resembles a Greek tragedy where the hero struggles against fate; or a World Series game with the pitcher preparing to throw the ball while the stadium audience, that classic chorus, roars mercilessly: "Let's go, let's go! What's the matter!" This, too, is the voice of the surgeon, for the contemporary surgeon who races from one hospital to another, from a hernia to a pilonidal cyst and on to a stomach, cannot afford to lose ten minutes for induction and preparation of his case—or so it seems to him. He cannot understand why one induction takes five minutes and the next, perhaps, five times as long.

If one asked this surgeon how he would like the ideal anesthesiologist to behave, he would probably answer somewhat along these lines: "As a matter of fact I prefer a nurse anesthetist.

But if I have to work with an anesthesiologist he should not be seen, heard, or in any other way noticeable."

Indeed, it is ideal if the anesthetist's performance does not attract anybody's attention. In the easy, good-risk cases this is often achieved. But, like the surgeon who cannot find the common duct because of anatomical anomalies, the anesthesiologist sometimes also encounters difficulties. He does the best he can with the anatomical and physiological material furnished by the patient. If the cards dealt you include aces and kings, you easily win the rubber; if there are no honors, you go down. In this case, the art consists in losing as little as possible.

After an easy, uneventful procedure, the surgeon may compliment the anesthesiologist; after a difficult case with ups and downs, in which the patient was nevertheless pulled through, the surgeon complains. And yet it is in the latter instance that the anesthetist demonstrates to the full his experience, judgment, and skill. So it is in retreat that a general demonstrates his talents and endurance. But the general has help—subordinates, assistants, chiefs of staff—while the anesthesiologist is alone: Between him and the failing patient there is no one (perhaps only a prayer).

II

It is the nature of anesthesia to strip the patient biologically and to put him through different antecedent stages of evolution. First, in the classic case, the spinal cord is affected and reflexes are exaggerated before they are cut down; then the cortex is irritated (hallucinations) prior to being completely switched off (unconsciousness); finally, cardiac and respiratory centers are approached. The patient, reversing as it were his phylogenetic stages—from human back to vertebrate and ameba—may manifest himself in primitive forms, resembling, in succession, an anthropoid, a rodent, a fish, a mollusc, a vegetation. This is, when racial, constitutional, genetic factors come to the fore, checked only perhaps by acquired and firmly established cultural and educational patterns. Lacking these, we have before us

on the operating table what is, in great part, a result of physiological and phylogenetic factors. This crude material reacts differently in varying races, nations, and social strata.

There are patients whose throat and larynx should not be
touched in the light phase of anesthesia: they will go into violent
laryngeal spasm. Others cannot be tubed readily with our Western laryngoscopes and tubes: their jaws and tongues weigh more
than expected—or so it seems; it can even be impossible to put
such patients correctly onto the operating table—their frames
simply do not fit. In short, knocked out, unconscious, left biologically naked on the table, the patients present differences in a
variety of acquired and inborn traits. These group particularities
have yet to find a reflection in our literature.

While the patient is undergoing changes due to narcosis, the
surgeon and the anesthesiologist may also demonstrate new, surprising aspects: under situations of specific stress this occurs
frequently. The anesthesiologist suddenly discloses his other,
underlying constitution and to everyone's surprise manifests a
decided lack of courage. The same may be true of the surgeon:
the great contemporary hero, the bully, the prima donna, suddenly loses his head and calls for a doctor in the house. There is
in surgical procedure the moment of truth, exactly as in the
corrida. An anesthesiologist or a surgeon who has once lost a
child on the operating table often can be recognized, like a toreador who has previously been gored. During the preliminaries,
he does everything as he used to, as custom and accepted technique ordain. But at the decisive moment, when the "kill" must
be performed, the man seems frightened, frozen, paralyzed, and
the arena understands: he is through, he must quit or he will be
killed. And he either quits or gets killed. This is the toreador's
case.

The case of anesthetist and surgeon is different: Next morning you see them again. At this stage of the game they never
voluntarily quit. Since it is usually not the physician who expires
in the operating room, they continue for several years their inadequate and disturbing activity. We all have seen such
"wounded" doctors; they are characterized by exaggerated reaction during a sudden complication. The slightest danger and
they are on the verge of hysterical collapse—something akin to

combat fatigue. Of course, the patient too when brought into the operating room may control himself, comport himself with dignity, in a civilized way, or go completely to pieces in panic and hysteria—despite premedication.

Thus, in the operating room, we can always distinguish the worthy man from the pseudo-hero, the bully, the humbug. This holds true—in differing degrees and for different reasons—for patient, surgeon, and anesthesiologist.

III

The attitude of the patient who is faced with an operation is undoubtedly important and may influence the outcome. It is one thing to induce anesthesia in a patient who is aware of the human condition, who accepts a reasonable amount of suffering as normal, and feels obliged and grateful to somebody in this world; it is quite another thing to handle a patient who thinks that nature owes him a pleasant life—without any vestige of pain—and who defends himself violently. Those can be two different kinds of anesthesia, often with very different biological and psychological results. Attitudes are different, reactions are different, the play of reflexes is different. It seems that the general culture of the patient, his beliefs and his philosophy, become an integral part of his organic life and exert a certain influence upon his physiology.

In this connection it is well to remember that our biological defense mechanisms have a salutary effect only up to a point, after which they may lead to disaster. In many instances, these personal self-defense systems, if excessively strong and stubborn, become the very cause of compensatory failure and death. Anyone who has ever tried to save a person from drowning knows what a nuisance the so-called instinct of self-preservation is; should the latter have its own way, both the drowning man and his rescuer would go down to the bottom.

The more a patient bleeds, the more defensive vasoconstriction is induced; his failing system, however, does not have the functional resources to overcome the increasing resistance and to pump the blood into the vital organs through those narrowed vessels. The paradox is that it would be better for the patient if his defense mechanism were weaker. "Therefore it is more expedient, at some stages of dying and resuscitation, to weaken the resistance of an organism, to lower the level of its vital activity."[1]

This vital activity depends on the interrelation of the vegetative reflexes—still an unexplored phenomenon. We routinely speak of separate vital reflexes, while it is their *interplay* that makes up the vital phenomenon and is responsible for most of the fatal accidents in the operating room. In the mind of the layman, anesthesia stands for suppression of pain. But this does not tell us much, since we lack a definition of pain (however concrete the notion itself may be). Furthermore, anesthesia does not abolish pain but only postpones it. (Here, again, the strange role of time in anesthesia manifests itself.) The patient may suffer later, when the surgeon has accomplished his job and left the premises. In fact, the surgeon would not mind operating on a patient who, while suffering agonies, could control his defense reflexes, not contract his belly and refrain from kicking the doctor in the groin. (In the Far East, where ancient disciplines are still practiced, certain operations and reductions of the joints are performed without interference of drugs and gases.)

Thus anesthesia is, first of all, the abolishment of the patient's defense mechanism—exposing him, unprotected, on the operating table. By doing this, the anesthesiologist must, accordingly, himself assume the defense of the patient against all potential dangers, even if this danger is personified by the overly radical surgeon.

The modern machines for respiration combined with intubation (which indeed assure perfect relaxation) lull us into a sense of false security; very often, patients are brought into complete apnea under the pretext of "better control"—whatever this may mean. To control the respiration in an emergency or for a short period, for the convenience of the exploring surgeon, is no doubt indicated; to "control" for hours and hours, almost inevitably overloading heart and lungs, seems sheer madness.

This tendency to control the patient goes even further. Due to new hypotensive and hypothermic techniques and the success of cardiac massage, there is now a trend to "control" the heart itself, to markedly slow down the rate of contraction or stop it completely for a while. This practice started in cardiac surgery and is now moving on to more banal procedures. We can almost envisage voluntary cardiac arrest for a hemorrhoidectomy or an abortion; it's not being done yet but the trend is there.

Granted that in some cases and for a short duration the procedure may be indicated and even lifesaving, this method of "control" brings us to a general problem: What does "to control" mean? Should the patient be controlled? Is it permissible for medicine or anesthesia so intimately and indiscriminately to interfere with the most vital processes of a human being—without our knowing all the pros and cons of such interference?

There are cultures that recognize the importance for the individual to control *his own* vital processes, cultures that carefully foster such control of the voluntary as well as the involuntary, vegetative systems. Alas, we Westerners have no part in this yet. And our attempts at delving into this field are sporadic and superficial. Instead, the researchers continue to bleed poor dogs, pump blood and oxygen back into them in their laboratories, so as to come up with the same dull reports that overlap and duplicate each other.

IV

The stress of administering anesthesia is in some instances so great that it could be compared to driving a heavy truck in bad weather. For this reason, the operating room is now swamped with electronic devices meant to assure safety. However, the simplest measures—known to all truck companies—have not been adopted: Stop at regular intervals, take a nap, drink a cup of coffee, rest!

Charles Lindbergh, flying the Atlantic, almost met with disaster: His fuel tank was nearly exhausted before he remembered to make the necessary switch to the second tank. He had no electronic devices! But Carpenter, whose capsule was filled with millions of dollars worth of electronic equipment, did not fare any better, as he, too, simply forgot, when preparing for descent, to shut off one system after he had already set in motion the other. He overshot his landing spot by two hundred miles, an error that might have resulted in disaster. In anesthesia, too, no electronic device can replace judgment, experience, and the constant check the "pilot" must keep up; how important that he not be overworked, frightened, or deadly tired.

It is accepted practice for an anesthetist to work as long as there are cases scheduled. If there is one case, he does one. If seven are booked, he performs them all—voluntarily, should he be billing for himself; under duress, if he is used by one of the numerous tycoon anesthesiologists. Should he be on call during the night, he may have to do an intestinal obstruction followed, perhaps, by a Cesarian section. Next morning, at a quarter to eight, he must start on the usual stomach, followed by several other cases; must handle needles, cyclopropane, halothane, curare, and other deadly weapons; register blood pressure, pulse, respiration, and all vital signs. That such routine can be, and in fact has been, a cause of disaster ought to be obvious to all parties concerned.

Having finished his second case on Long Island at 10:30 A.M., a surgeon rushes through heavy local traffic to a hernia in Brooklyn; at 12:30 he washes down a sandwich with a cup of coffee and immediately begins a cholycystectomy. He cuts the hepatic artery, which is not in the usual place, or he even ties the common duct, while the anesthetist, pumping the sixth unit of blood and simultaneously pressing the oxygen bag, notices at that very moment that the curare-like solution is still dripping into the vein. Or a sponge is missing—and X-rays show that it has been left in the patient's belly. What of this is due to "natural causes," and therefore part of the calculated risk, and what to simple human fatigue, overextension of physical and spiritual faculties? Perhaps surgeon and anesthetist should take at least the same precautions as a truck driver?

Countess Alexandra Tolstoi tells in her memoirs of the hysterectomy a famous surgeon performed on her mother. From Tula or Moscow he came, with equipment and nurses, to their estate, Yasnaya Polyana. For a day or two, the entire suite of rooms was scrubbed, soaped, washed. The professor operated slowly (a subtotal, I bet); after successfully closing up, he felt so weak from exhaustion or excitement that he began to shake, exactly as a singer or pianist might after a great concert performance. He sipped a glass of champagne and went to bed—at noon!

Well, this is perhaps a bit too much, even for a Chaliapin. But—on the other hand—to start out from Westchester at a quarter to seven with the traffic, come through it victoriously, enter the elevator at 8:15 and "let's go, come on now, how long is it going to take you to put the patient to sleep. . . ."? The surgeon's schedule: one stomach, two hernias, a pilonidal cyst, and a frozen section—all this at two or perhaps three different hospitals. The pilonidal cyst turns out to be infected; consequently there is no clean room available for the next case—and he was late to begin with. All this is not as it should be. But he is the patron of the hospital, and the patron is always right.

The anesthesiologist who conscientiously makes his rounds, the night before, to study the patient is met with incomplete charts, no physical, no history, no lab report as yet, and frustrating statements from the ignorant patient. "Doctor, I do not want a spinal"; or "Doctor, I do not want ether"; "I do not want a mask on my face"; "I was promised only a needle in the vein—nothing more"; and many other equally silly demands.

The present-day man fancies himself a very sophisticated fellow. He has read articles in the *Readers Digest*. He knows that cancer is cured, by isotopes or radical surgery or both, in 87 percent of the cases. He is certain it was the spinal that caused his mother-in-law's terrible headache . . . but he is ignorant of the simple fact that 8:00 A.M. is the best time for an elective operation.

An operation is in many ways like a boxing match; the more rounds, the more exhausted are the challengers. Also, the more cases that have been performed, the more microorganisms have accumulated in the operating room. On his own, the patient cannot realize this. He needs to be educated. Should he find out about the drawbacks of a routine where several major operations are performed in one day by the same man, perhaps that practice would soon end. So far, on the contrary, the patient feels proud that his surgeon is such a busy man. As for being without food or *water* for eighteen hours until the operation—that he thinks is not important.

V

To practice modern medicine among the bushmen, it is not enough to bring in modern equipment, electronic devices, laboratories, and medical personnel. The problem is to educate the people, so that they know when to seek medical help, know the nature of that help, learn what to expect and what not to expect of a doctor, and, above all, what to ask of themselves.

An acquaintance of mine, appointed superintendent of a hospital in central Australia, upon his arrival there eagerly asked one of the doctors: "Tell me, how does medicine function here?"

"Come with me to the office and see for yourself," the doctor replied.

An elderly, almost naked, rather emaciated native walked in, pointing to his stomach. The doctor quickly examined him, wrote out a prescription, and told him to have it filled at the dispensary. The old man walked out.

"Now come with me," the doctor said to the superintendent.

They followed the old man through backyards to his hut and watched him bend over a fire, take up some embers in an iron dish, and carefully burn the prescription; after which he collected the ashes, chewed them up thoroughly, and washed them down with a gulp of water. When the newcomer looked at the doctor in dismay, the latter said: "Don't feel so bad. Can't you see, we are already halfway there!"

Obviously, modern medicine cannot be applied under such conditions. Unless the natives are also reeducated in all other respects, modern practices of medicine will remain hocus-pocus and magic.

The same applies to our natives here. Unless they learn what medicine can and cannot be; unless they recognize the meaning of growth, maturity, old age; unless they come to accept pain, in principle, medical practice here and everywhere will bear the same stigmata as in central Australia.

Polar explorers speak of the warming up of the arctic. Indeed, during the last seventy-five years, a rise in temperature at both poles has been observed, and life and agriculture have become possible in regions where formerly they could not develop. Similarly, other peculiar changes have taken place in the last decades. One of them appears to be a softening of human nature.

History and ethnology tell us how people, from early, so-called primitive societies up, endured privations, pain, torture, and agony. The code of behavior, from commoner to nobleman, imposed certain rules that no threats, fear, or torture could influence. It is not like that any more. Call it brainwashing, or softness, or plain cowardice; the fact is that even superior officers have, the day after falling into the hands of the enemy, confessed any guilt, individual or collective; divulged all secrets, real or imaginary; retracted their statements, reasserted them, and made any compromise rather than face pain or the fear of pain.

The postoperative patient clamoring for needles and pills is only one symptom of a widespread condition of compromise and softening that dominates contemporary life. Our era considers pain and suffering the supreme evil. But the very fear of pain and suffering has assumed such proportions that it now distorts our entire life, resulting in a culture where each seeks, above all, pleasure—pleasure and comfort for himself.

The fight against the "population explosion," the search for oral contraceptives, unrestricted abortions, and multiple orgasms, are basically outcomes of the same trend: comfort above all—here and now.

Of course, a stoic approach to pain and discomfort—what William James calls "the athletic attitude of the soul"—does not begin and end in the doctor's office, the hospital, or the operating room; our attitude toward pain and discomfort covers a much wider range and may well be the key to many contemporary ills.

Anesthesiology, concerned as it is with human beings under stress and with their vital responses and resistance, is by its very nature called to play a role in the development of a new attitude toward stimuli and pain. Pain is not useless; pain has a meaning; life implies a measure of pain and suffering. Our human dignity lies in accepting and overcoming them, up to a point—by free choice and in good spirit. This is a religious approach, one that has been discarded in favor of a naive faith in fictitious science and automatic progress.

VI

One of the pillars of this fictitious science is *statistics*. As all statistics dealing with small series, medical statistics are open to extensive interpretation. And this makes them a highly subjective matter. To consider the field of statistics an exact science is just as preposterous as to consider history one. There is no history, there are only historians! According to some, the French Revolution was an evil; according to others it was the salvation of mankind. Of statistics, too, it can be said: There are no statistics, there are only statisticians! And in the medical-biological field with its limited amount of cases and unlimited participating elements—many of them completely unknown—the statisticians are at least as handicapped as the historians.

The elements that can influence a human organism are innumerable. However, we take into consideration only those elements that we have postulated as valid. Just one "silly" example: It was never seriously considered whether the relation of the sleeping body to the earth's axis (and the magnetic field) might be of any importance in the etiology of cancer. Should we have to include this element, all previous statistical elaborations would become null and void. And such possible causes can be put forward *ad infinitum*.

Recently some extraordinary statistics, based on 6,800 births, indicated that neonatal mortality for premature infants born to nonsmoking mothers is about double that for premature infants born to smoking mothers.[2] Are such elaborations not rather futile?

Furthermore, it is well to realize that in certain fields, and anesthesia is one of them, the charts on which statistics are based are, for the most part, false or falsified; and the most dramatic, truly significant, and instructive cases (with shock, collapse, resuscitation) are precisely the ones that are poorly recorded. In a dramatic incident, the anesthesiologist—usually alone—must simultaneously pump oxygen and blood, check the pulse, inject a stimulant; and usually it is at this very point that the infusion begins to infiltrate or the pint of blood is knocked down by a harried nurse.

"Is my tube in place?" "Was the suction catheter far enough?" "Is the patient light or deep?" "Is his heart beating or not?" These are some of the questions that race through the anesthetist's mind at such moments when it seems almost impossible for one person in, so to say, no time, to check and control all aspects of the situation.

But afterwards you read the chart, and you see that the blood pressure was checked every five minutes (systolic and diastolic); so was the pulse; ephedrin was injected at precisely 9:24; levophed at 9:48; the second pint of blood suspended at 10:00 A.M. on the dot; blood pressure rose exactly one minute after administration of ACTH. How did we arrive at such a picture?

If the drama lasted approximately twenty-five minutes, the anesthetist divides this interval later into stages of spontaneous, assisted, and controlled respiration; normal blood pressure, lowered blood pressure, and systolic 40mm Hg; then cardiac massage, defibrillation; and so on, and so on.

Mark Twain said that "in real life the thing never happens at the right place, at the right time: it is the business of the historian to remedy this mistake." Not *only* of the historian!

This procedure would not be so fraught with error under normal conditions. But we already noted how strangely time changes in connection with anesthesia. Those "two minutes" of cardiac arrest can, depending on the depth of anesthesia and the patient's temperature and metabolism, be equivalent to five minutes or five seconds.

According to Einstein's special theory of relativity, time has no absolute meaning; under high velocity it shrinks—so that the twin brother who went for a ride in cosmic space for a couple of decades would return younger than the one who stayed all that time in New York City, minding his own business. Biologically it can mean only one thing: High velocity slows down the metabolic rate, and, in anesthesia hypothermia and hypotension, conserves the organism longer.

Of course under stress, time changes its flow also for anesthetist and surgeon.

Considering all this, it is pure fantasy to divide a critical period in the operating room into several definite, logical parts. Despite all the good will of the anesthesiologist, his record must turn out to be fictional if not without a certain artistic value. Looking at those curves, threads, circles, dots and figures, hurriedly agglomerated across the chart and diluted with sweat, blood, and vomit, a man with some imagination can well realize that here, on a sheet of paper representing the span of barely one hour and a half, a battle with an eternal meaning was faintly recorded and that highly specialized men tried to apply the best of their knowledge, skill, and wisdom (even if lacking the opportunity to note down, at the precise moments, their doings and undoings).

But from a scientific point of view such charts are of no use, even if they do not accumulate conscious lies and omissions. The more rational and unequivocal, the cleaner the chart, the falser it is! Dramas are not logical—yet our charts, *nolens volens*, follow the cause-and-effect dictum.

Similar aspects must prevail in other fields whenever the past is recorded from a position occupied later, establishing the cause, so to say, only after the effect has shown up. Such information is false (or partially false) and therefore worse than no information at all.

VII

It is the general trend in contemporary surgery to consider even radical surgical interference as "a trifle." The advent of antibiotics, anesthesia, electrolyte and fluid balance, supposedly has turned surgery into an everyday procedure. "In a week or so you will be home and forget the entire affair!"

The surgeon usually claims that his patient—a cancer of the stomach or the lung—"has a chance only if we operate immediately." The anesthesiologist may differ in the evaluation; he may feel that in this particular case there is not even the claimed five to ten percent curative chance. "If the good Lord wants him to die, let him die without my interference," he thinks. As a medical specialist with broad experience in surgical cases and acquainted with a variety of surgeons of different schools, the anesthesiologist cannot ignore his own judgment, especially in the case of poor-risk patients.

In such instances he is faced with a moral issue. He does not approve of this particular operation on this particular patient at this particular time. It is against his accumulated experience and philosophy. Yet, under the pretext that it is the surgeon who is responsible for *everything* that goes on in the operating room, the anesthesiologist administers anesthesia.

And this is wrong! For he, too, is a physician, in the broadest sense of this word, and he takes part in a procedure he considers useless, perhaps fatal. To deny his personal responsibility makes him akin to the guard of a concentration camp who denies his guilt under the pretext that he acted on orders of his "superiors."

If the specialization of physicians in the field of anesthesia is here to stay, the trained anesthesiologist must have a voice not only in the choice and conduct of anesthesia but also in the decision as to whether a particular patient should be operated on at that particular time, at that particular hospital. Otherwise, such medical specialization does not make sense. "To give anesthesia is not difficult; but to give safe anesthesia is."[3] This can only mean that, often, the anesthesiologist must postpone a case or refuse it altogether.

The classical legal comparison of the surgeon with the captain of a ship is absurd. It can only be explained by the fact that the judges also have their problems, that they too indulge in outdated notions about medicine and, above all, are also looking for a single authority or, rather, a hero. There is no drama without a hero, and there is no hero if there are two heroes. Any Hollywood producer knows this. The court must have felt the same way. This of course flatters the surgeon's ego. Perhaps this is why he prefers a nurse anesthetist at the head of the table to a physician with broad education and training.

The captain of a ship sinks with his ship. If he gets off, he is the last to leave; otherwise he has a hard time explaining it. This is not the case of the surgeon: The patient may die but the captain goes on to the next operating room.

The captain of a ship receives from his superiors an order in a sealed envelope and makes off for the seven seas. He may have a secret mission and, despite the engineer's warning that the boiler will explode, he orders to increase speed; somewhere, far off, sinking with his ship, he can radio: mission accomplished.

Well, in the operating room there can be no secret missions and no diverting maneuvers; everybody knows what he is there for, and if the ship sinks—if the patient dies—it is obvious that the mission was *not* accomplished.

The supremacy of the surgeon degrades the other medical specialists in the operating room, particularly the anesthesiologist who is far too often expected to act against his own judgment. That, in a matter of mutual concern, the judgment of one medical specialist should a priori prevail over the judgment of another medical specialist is metaphysically wrong and factually harmful.

Part II
SURGERY

Surgery is irreversible

I

As in many a fairy tale, the hero of our story has a humble beginning. Once there was a barber. He was so clever with his hands, shaving, massaging neck and scalp, excising calluses in the public baths, that the medical man took to calling in the barber when he needed some skilful manipulations with a limb or wanted a patient bled.

Such is the origin of our hero. From here he worked his way up. You may verily say he is a self-made man. Still and all, until the 19th century, his role remained ambiguous and dependent upon the medical doctor.

The surgeon has come a long way since: he has studied anatomy, pathology, even some physiology; instead of "mister" he became "doctor," which is only just. But then, something Freudian or Adlerian occurred. Recalling his background and historical past, the former barber decided, consciously or unconsciously, to get even with the medical man and to steal the show.

Where is the old darling doctor, Pasteurian beard and all, rushing through the night in his buggy with a supply of powders and elixirs for the dying woman or the babe burning up in fever? He whips his horse on as he murmurs: "If only I can arrive in time (with my powder and pills!)." Where is this hero of the past? He is gone! Where is the bacteriologist, navigating on the seas, penetrating into the jungle, test tube in hand, in quest of unknown microorganisms? This hero, too, has vanished. And neither did the pathologist quite make the grade.

The hero of our present-day fairy tales, of the movies, TV, newspaper reports, schools, and, of course, the hospitals is the surgeon. He is the superman of the medical profession, the god who possesses the power of restoration and salvation.

Does such a myth correspond with reality? Is this myth of value to the patient and society? These are the questions we pose. They are important questions, for we believe that surgery is, at the present time, running amok; has long stepped out of its indicated boundaries; has changed from a limited, beneficial service into a gigantic, distorted monstrosity.

Strangely enough, this distortion is not caused by some unscrupulous, dishonest, cynical individuals but by the idealistic, ambitious fanatics of surgery, and therefore it can be corrected only if the entire philosophy of surgery is revised from the roots and new principles are established.

II

It is common knowledge that unhappy people often seek refuge in sickness. Some of these confused and disturbed ones land with the psychoanalyst. But many neurotics—and this fact is not so well known—crowd the surgeon's office. They undergo one operation after another, they insist on them; for thus they find for a while relief from their depression—exactly as after shock treatment. This is a relatively new phenomenon, fostered by a society that seeks immediate, tangible results—and by the corresponding radical trend in surgery.

There are surgeons who tell their patients that all hernias should be repaired and all fibroids excised (preferably together with the uterus); there are surgeons who claim that *repeat* Cesarian sections are always justified and that cancer of the breast has a 75 percent five-year survival rate after radical mastectomy (and much less after simple). All such surgeons are dangerous fanatics.

Public opinion should be aroused against their extremist doctrines. The patient should be made aware that there are almost always two schools of thought, and that both are equally justified on the basis of our present state of knowledge (or ignorance). The fact is that not every hernia need be operated; that not every fibromatous uterus is useless (not even after menopause); that repeat section is not, a priori, imperative; and, first of all and above all, that radical surgery is no solution to cancer.

The surgeon should tell the patient that some doctors believe in his way of treatment but that others, also good ones, would not operate in this particular case, or would perform only a simple procedure. The patient would have to take part in the—for him—so vital discussion of the pros and cons. Even if he had to devote several weeks to gathering information, his time would not be wasted, for major surgery is an *irreversible* process.

III

One of the reasons for surgical aggressiveness is our fetish for "playing it safe."

Here is a boy of nine with right lower abdominal pain. Should he be operated on immediately for possible appendicitis or not? The play-it-safe principle decides—often against better judgment. Should a baby with *possible* open inguinal ring be operated on for a hernia? Should we take out one kidney, the spleen, the gallbladder, uterus, prostate, three quarters of the stomach, both breasts, both ovaries, both tonsils, at some vague, suspicion-arousing indications? Does this really mean to "play it safe"? Are the tonsils completely useless, does the uterus become obsolete after childbearing, does any stone in the gallbladder render it superfluous—and will the cholecystectomy solve all the problems?

The general trend in modern medicine is such that soon, thanks to the combination of the "play-safe" principle and the drive of the surgeons who are running amok, every living body in all the well-to-do countries will have been mutilated, regardless of race, creed, or social status.

Here is a typical example of such modern aspirations: "While removal of the appendix when the abdomen is opened for other reasons is not only condoned but is urged as good practice, and while a few attacks of tonsillitis are taken as ample justification for tonsillectomy, hysterectomy is deplored unless there is no other method of handling the problem at hand. It is about this special status of the uterus that we must have a change of attitude in view of our changed knowledge and skills. 'Except for the childbearing function, the uterus is a dispensable organ. Not only can a woman get along satisfactorily without it, but without it she is free of certain nuisances and dangers.' "[4]

What exactly does it mean "to play safe"? Is the surgeon in a position to do it? And what kind of safe play does he have in mind? In order to understand what is safe and what unsafe, we have to realize all the pros and cons of our human condition from beginning to end (and, perhaps, farther). After all, to grow is a risky adventure; it might be safer to freeze on fetus level. A paramecium is practically immortal!

In a religious community, playing safe means to be in communion with God and one's neighbor; this insures everlasting life and happiness. For a Marxist, to play safe is to join the growing forces of the leading historical class.

But what is playing safe for the contemporary middle-class agnostic? He is not certain about God; he dislikes metaphysics; he does not trust the mechanic at the garage and the policeman on the beat; he does not believe his lawyer or his congressman. He knows that everything around him is rotten, crooked, bribed, and blackmailed. He seeks facts, and checks and rechecks all available data. Yet, if his doctor tells him that in order to "play safe" he should have his gallbladder removed, he lands sheepishly, without further discussion, on the operating table. Because from childhood on he has been hypnotized by the idea of the infallibility of science—and he has been told that medicine is a science!

Well, it is time to inform our man that this is not so; that even in such disciplines as physics and mathematics the contemporary trend is to deny the possibility of precise, objective knowledge. Planck expressed doubts along these lines, and the scientists who succeeded him in quantum mechanics went further along this path. We know now that it is impossible to find out both the energy and the position of a nuclear particle simultaneously. Our instruments of observation interfere and change either the position or the speed of the particle—without any possible correction. Thus, reality is indeterminable.[5] If indetermination and lack of information are introduced into higher physics, how much more a factor are they then in biology and physiology and internal medicine!

Here it is perhaps fitting to divulge a secret which is somehow forgotten by the average physician. The fact is that there is *not one* medical test that is one hundred percent specific! There are, for instance, eighty diseases that will give a false positive reaction for syphilis. And the same is the case for all other laboratory results (not counting human error). The pathology results on cancer, also, are not absolute: not absolute either *for* or *against*.

IV

Garage mechanics will replace generators, batteries, carburetors, radiators, at random, until they sometimes hit upon the real cause of trouble. This revolts us. Many people familiarize themselves with the car engine so as not to be at the mercy of incompetent and/or unscrupulous service-station workers. These people do not wish to be "suckers."

Doctors, lawyers, engineers, are all human. Education and college degree do not vouchsafe honesty and proper conduct. If it were otherwise, there would be a marked decrease in the number of crooks with the increase in college degrees. There are as many amoral people in the medical profession as in other trades and occupations. All people must choose between good and evil, and this is as difficult for a doctor as for an automobile mechanic. Yet in all other fields, the common man is prepared to defend himself; in the matter of medical care he becomes an easy prey. He was conditioned to *believe* in science. What is more, he would not even have the criteria by which to judge a doctor; what he does and does not like about a physician is really of no great importance: the bedside manner, the professional look, the expensive car. . . .

It is a well-established fact that a sort of platonic love affair takes place between patient and psychoanalyst during a certain period of the treatment. Something on the manner of this "transference" exists between many patients and their physicians. It would be sheer madness to ask the psychoanalyst to take out your child's tonsils; but this is exactly what many a thankful mother asks the family doctor who delivered the child to do.

How often does one hear the name of a surgeon or

gynecologist mentioned with reverence, while those who have seen him in the operating room question his abilities. Naive evaluations are made not only by laymen but even by general practitioners, endocrinologists, radiologists, and other specialists who do not frequent the operating room.

People hate to be cheated where it concerns a shock absorber, but in the most important matters concerning their own life they submit with complete ignorance to mere appearances. The problem is obviously an educational one.

Here we are not after the unscrupulous surgeon or gynecologist; the law or the medical societies will eventually catch up with him. The real danger is the good, honest surgeon; the radical surgeon who *believes* in surgery, who loves to operate; the crusader who thinks that he can save humanity with his scalpel.

Should he be right, then everything is in its place and we ought to submit to twenty million operations a year (not counting those under local anesthesia). But should he be wrong, then we are confronted with a terrible amount of needless suffering and a fantastic waste of life and money.

V

According to some medical statistics (all of which are inclined to be rather optimistic), only 10 percent of lung cancer patients "survive" five years after radical surgery. This survival may of course be due to other processes and not to the radical operation! On the other hand, the lives of a great number of such patients are shortened by radical surgery. For these cases no relative statistics are available. Is it worth going through the torture—and expense—of such an operation for a 10 percent chance of "cure" (five years survival) as against an n percent chance of actually having one's life shortened? This is the sort of question one can only answer *for oneself*.

In our civilization, the mature citizen of good standing is supposed to have an opinion about political affairs—so as to be fit to vote; he must know some basic theology—so as to understand why he goes to his particular church and not to the one across the street; he learns to distinguish between noises from a rotten exhaust pipe and inadequate pistons; he even knows that he prefers Mozart to Wagner or Titian to Picasso. Why not, then, a more critical approach to medicine, for no one will defend your entity the way you would do it yourself.

Plato states in his *Republic*: "And yet what greater proof can there be of a bad and disgraceful state of education than this, that not only the artisans and the meaner sort of people need the skill of first-rate physicians and judges, but also those who would profess to have had a liberal education? Is it not disgraceful and a great sign of want of good-breeding, that a man should have to go abroad for his law and physic because he has none of his own at home, and must therefore surrender himself into the hands of other men whom he makes lords and judges over him?"

His foe Aristotle once said to the physician who was giving him instructions: "Do not treat me like a shepherd or a ploughman. First of all, explain why you advise it; then I am ready to obey."

This is how the ailing Freud defined his essential demands for the patient-doctor relationship: "But first he wanted a basic understanding to be reached on the conditions for such a relationship. He expressed the expectation that he would always be told the truth and nothing but the truth. My response must have reassured him that I meant to keep such a promise."[6]

Of course, not everybody writes the *Dialogues* or invents psychoanalysis but, strangely enough, if left alone and not "conditioned," many of us would feel more or less the way Plato and Freud felt about medicine.

In a civilized society the patient should be educated enough to take part in the deliberations about a radical intervention or an aggressive cure and—with family doctor, specialist, and relatives—weigh the pros and cons. The last decision must be his, in accordance with his general outlook, preferences, philosophy, and faith. No surgeon, however great, however much the superman, however honored, wealthy, and admired, can make this decision for somebody else. If and when the surgeon himself has to go through a pneumonectomy, then, of course, only he himself has the right to make the decision. But only then. (And many a specialist has told me that he would never submit to a major operation in his particular field—unless his life, socially and professionally, had become unbearable.) The so-called *facts* of science, the so-called facts of statistics, are actually matters of interpretation, which different individuals with different philosophies interpret differently.

VI

It is perhaps comforting to pay a sum of money and delegate the burden of a decision to someone else, but in vital matters such as marriage, religion, career, personal health, and survival it is sheer madness.

If we could for a moment forget the training and conditioning we received from childhood, would it not seem madness to permit a man, who knows a certain technique and has a state license, to cut you with knife or scalpel any time he chooses and at any particular spot, without your personally checking and rechecking his verdict? Should not some precautions of a general and deeper nature be taken?

By distorting the proportions, a little truth becomes a big lie. Contemporary medicine, in which radical interventions play such an inordinate role, is such a distortion of the truth. It's only human to exaggerate one's own importance: Psychoanalysts claim that most pathologies have their origin in infantile complexes; the chiropractor *knows* that any disturbance in the human body is due to a bend in the spinal vertebrae, and he is ready to cure the entire scale of abnormalities, from mental disturbances to cancer of the blood, by manipulation of the spine; the podiatrist believes that corns and calluses throw the individual off balance and become the source of innumerable complications. Is it surprising that the surgeon, too, exaggerates his role in the medical economy and has his 100 percent cure that consists of repeated, total, "radical" extirpations? I know of doctors who constantly run through public and private schools to pick out children with possible open inguinal rings, whom they then pass on to the surgeon. According to the now-prevailing philosophy they act in good faith and are justified. No medical society will condemn them.

Every hospital that wishes to be respectable boasts a so-called tissue committee that checks on the specimens removed by surgery. But this does not solve our problem, since these committees do not question the established contemporary philosophy according to which the presence of a fibroid justifies hysterectomy and a microscopical examination of the removed specimen showing inflamation gives, post factum, the green light for removal of the gallbladder. Nor do they question repeated surgery on sufferers from progressive diseases such as degenerative arthritis and vascular insufficiency. (Thus surgeons operate every year on the same victim, till death them do part.) What we seek is a change in the philosophy of surgery, so that such operations will not, automatically, be considered good practice.

In addition there are surgical interventions where specimens cannot be expected, for instance the diaphragmatic hernias. Those operations are the real bread and butter of the ambitious surgeon, and no one can check on him in these cases, for there is no excised specimen to examine.

VII

The notion of an operation as "a trifle"—the patient gets a needle in the vein, falls asleep, awakens, and a week later leaves the hospital—this notion, even though reality often seems to conform to it, is a dangerous lie. But thus it is usually presented, for the general trend is to operate—to operate early, and often, and more and more radically.

The gynecologist, to demonstrate his superior specialization, never takes out only the uterus but grabs the cervix as well. This is the total hysterectomy! Even supposing any fibroid did justify hysterectomy, why take out the cervix as well, thus doubling operating time and risks, and mutilating the vagina? The philosophy behind it is to avoid the risk of possible carcinoma of the cervix. This way we play safe! On the other hand, any conscientious gynecologist who performs a total hysterectomy on a woman not yet in menopause leaves tubes and ovaries at least partially intact, if they are not diseased. And yet, carcinoma of the ovaries, too, is a reality (in some races proportionally higher than carcinoma of the cervix).

Is there any consistency in such a practice, for which the patient pays bodily and materially: vagina completely void of contents, sexual life impoverished, support for bladder and rectum substantially diminished, if not null. And before she knows what is happening, a cystocele and a rectocele develop, the gynecologist again establishes himself on the stool, in front of the patient with her legs raised and spread, and now a vaginal plastic is performed—to the full satisfaction of all parties involved, since Blue Cross coverage makes it seem a free gift to the patient. All this is done in good faith and according to the best medical standards. Not the men are to blame but the philosophy that backs them up.

There is growing evidence that in most instances of cancer the results of radical or simple intervention are the same. This seems to refute common sense, but physiology, biology, life, and science are not based on common sense. Perhaps some *uncommon sense* would help us more. Medical authorities are steadily becoming more aware of the fact that radical surgery is no answer to cancer. Still, the torture does not stop, for there is, as yet, nothing to replace it.

On the other hand there is the fact that clinical observation definitely demonstrates a self-defense against cancer. The phenomenon of spontaneous regression of metastases after limited removal of the primary tumor is a mysterious but established fact. Some attribute these cures to the reticuloendothelial system; other immunological processes may also be involved in such regressions. With cruel surgical and X-ray interference we attack, from without, not only the tumor but also those salutary immunological processes as well.

"The possibility that reduced resistance due to extensive surgery or high-dose roentgen therapy for cancer may have an accelerating effect on metastasis has been suggested by a researcher here on the basis of experiments . . . Dr. Kallenbeck said . . . these laboratory experiments raise some important questions about the clinical treatment of cancer patients. Improved techniques in cancer therapy have enabled us to remove ever larger tumors and make more progress in preventing local recidivistic tendencies. But it seems to me the time may have come to examine whether these radical treatments don't reduce the patient's resistance and endanger the ultimate goal of therapy—the patient's recovery."[7]

Massive stress and trauma defeat the purpose of the operation. But the ambitious surgeon cannot resign himself to a secondary role; he multiplies, increases, deepens the interventions, ad absurdum. In cancer of the breast, for instance, the result of mastectomy, whether simple or radical, is the same—a very poor one. It is much poorer than official statistics—which, incidentally, do not consider those patients whose life was shortened by radical procedures (during and after operation)—claim. Furthermore, these statistics are based solely on the five years "survival" time and do not take into account that, already after the second year, in many cases metastases appear and the patient's life becomes a martyrdom due to repeated operations, poisonous X-ray treatment, chemical perfusions, and constant drugging. This morbid picture is officially called "cure," if only it can be carried on into the sixth year after initial operation.

Intelligent surgeons are aware of these enormous contradictions but dare not draw the logical conclusions. On the contrary, attempts are made to further radicalize the radical procedures: The ribs beneath the diseased breast are taken out, the surgeons arguing how best to close the mutilated thorax, and the patients dying from surgical trauma or, if they survive for a while, suffering inordinately. The philosophy is to extirpate the lymphatic system that runs along the ribs (and that is part of the immunogenic system!). But the lymphatic systems are connected; why not take out the one on the opposite side as well? And what about the para-vertebral chains? And if, by some miracle, we learn how to cut out the entire thorax—what about the circulatory system? For cancer is not only disseminated via lymph. Does it all make sense?

Behind it stands the ambitious surgeon with creative mind and dedicated soul. This is the evil. Perhaps he should be told that surgery just is not big enough for all his aspirations, that it is a limited field: for local intervention, to help other natural systems and biochemical processes gradually to restore the organism. Surgery is a palliation and as such should not be radical, and should not endanger or shorten the patient's life.

VIII

Here is a patient, let's call him General McArthur, eighty-four years old and exhibiting signs of jaundice. The papers do not give the details but it can be assumed that an X-ray of the gallbladder was taken and perhaps a stone or gravel visualized in the cystic or the common duct. Then the surgeons take over and, according to the papers, traumatize a man of eighty-four for three full hours. The operation is called a success; apparently the stone was removed and the common duct explored.

Seventeen days later they operate again. This time for a shunt, because of hypertension in the portal vein due to liver cirrhosis. A porta-caval or any other shunt on a postoperative, toxic patient of eighty-four is sheer madness. And why the first operation if, all along, it was hypertension of the portal vein? Is it not logical to assume that the liver cirrhosis existed already before the first operation—seventeen days ago—and that the jaundice could be attributed to it—and not to a gallstone? Exposure of an eighty-four-year-old patient to the useless first three-hour-long procedure may well have been the extra weight that tilted the precarious balance. Should, for reasons that escape the uninitiated, a drainage of the gallbladder have been indicated, why not stick in a catheter, i.e., why not perform a simple cholecystostomy, which would take such an expert team ten to fifteen minutes and could be performed under local anesthesia? But that would not be real surgery! The modern surgeon is trained to perform radical operations. A mere general practitioner can perform a cholecystostomy. For that you do not need a prima donna.

Here is the president of the United States. He feels discomfort after having eaten too many rich pies. X-rays show one little stone in the gallbladder. Cholecystectomy is advised and President Johnson meekly submits. During the operation a stone is discovered in the genito-urinary system—also on the right side!—and dug out. The question arises: Which stone gave the president his symptoms? Chances are that a physiologically healthy and still-functioning gallbladder was taken out. Paradoxically, a kidney stone on the left side was not removed, although it could not have been less pathological than the one on the right side. What a salient illustration for the misery of our medical sciences! And this was done to a man belonging to the very highest echelon. One can only guess at the abuse of radicalism rampant in the hospitals patronized by members of the middle classes.

That a radical trend in surgery is characteristic of the entire world, and not limited to this country, can be demonstrated by the case of the late king of Greece. Here we have a magnificent international team working for over three hours to perform a total or subtotal gastrectomy. Indication: peptic ulcer. A week or two later the king dies of an embolism.

Surgical trauma influences clotting time and coagulation; The incidence of emboli is in direct proportion to the time and scope of an operation. That is why we are against surgical trauma—unless necessary. Any textbook of physiology speaks of the hastening of blood coagulation in pain and great emotion. This is supposed to be a manifestation of an archaic defense mechanism (actually, any increase in the secretion of the adrenals, i.e., of the fighting spirit, has the same effect). The preoperative, operative, and postoperative periods are too critical periods of stress.[8]

Despite the so-called miraculous progress of surgery during the last decades, the amount of postoperative deaths is the *same*, percentage-wise, for the period from 1933–1943 and for the period from 1943–1960, notwithstanding blood transfusions, antibiotics, and wonder drugs! Only the primary causes have exchanged places. "Pyogenic infections decreased and moved from the second to the seventh place according to frequency. Peritonitis, for many years the primary cause of death, moved to fourth place. Pulmonary embolism increased and accounted for 14.5 percent of all postoperative deaths during this period."[9]

But our surgeon argues: "Everything went fine. I made such a good anastomosis. Is it my fault if the patient shoots an embolism in the second week?" Well, yes, it is your fault. This kind of stress and trauma was too much for the patient, even with the recent advances in medicine.

If the master team of surgeons working on the late king of Greece had remembered a simple procedure known as gastroen-terostomy (plus vagotomy), it would have taken them forty min-utes to operate and, again, this minimum stress might have tilted the scales in the favorable direction. But this would not have been radical surgery: A surgeon must be a superman, a hero, who, alone and radically, accomplishes the entire cure, here and now, leaving no doubt about his role in our lives.

Ironically, in this case it turned out not to be a simple peptic ulcer but a malignancy that, according to the more reliable statis-tics, has a "survival rate" of only 5 percent over five years. It is for these illusionary 5 percent that the tremendous procedure of total gastrectomy is quite often undertaken. If 5 percent do in-deed "survive" five years (while undergoing all manner of surgi-cal torture), the number of those whose life is drastically short-ened, as the king's, is certainly greater, but, in fact, unknown. Our medical statistics lean toward one direction. We get only two figures: One shows the five-year survival rate; the other shows those who did not reach that sacramental number. We are not told how many of the latter survived *less* than the probable life span of a cancer patient without aggressive surgery. Herein lies the mistake.

If we knew that the life span of 5 percent of the patients is prolonged, but that the life of, say, 45 percent is shortened, a new moral and legal problem would arise. Also, we must always bear in mind that to carry the patient for that five-year period of survival may demand new, painful, and costly interventions, which some patients, if well informed, would perhaps not wish to endure. Here should also be mentioned the king of England who, after a prolonged, mutilating pneumonectomy for cancer of the lung, finally died of embolism.

It was General Eisenhower's good fortune that he held the office of president of the United States at the time of his intesti-nal trouble. The team of first-class surgeons simply did not dare the radical procedure, since excision of the greater part of the small intestine presents an enormous risk. In ambitious surgery, the involved part of regional enteritis is excised. But in this case, so we heard, the radical method was abandoned in favor of a trivial bypass. Notice, it does make sense to excise the diseased toxic bowel; like everything else, it is a question of judgment and, the patient's life being involved, he too should know the pros and cons and take part in the final decision.

All these examples involve first-class, great, dedicated surgeons. But, as in any other profession, there also exist abuses by unscrupulous, immoral people. With a philosophy of preventive interventions, play-safe radicalism, and glorification of aggressive surgery to back them up, what can stop them—provided they have the paper qualifications?

IX

The psychoanalytic view of the surgeon as a sublimated butcher is a nearsighted glimpse of a larger truth. A closer knowledge of surgeons reveals many other sublimations: The barber is very much in evidence; so is the carpenter; and the plumber. And in the new fields of surgery we see the sublimated mechanic and the electrician at work. Indeed, many who overcrowd the operating room with machines and electronic gadgets seem to have been led astray from an MIT laboratory or the controls of a jet plane.

There also exist in this world cruel, strange, mad, men who like to cut and cut, to take apart and rebuild—like children who destroy a beautiful toy and then patch it up again. How interesting it must seem to this psychological type to open up a belly or a chest or even a heart, and then sew it up again. This kind of mania cannot be forbidden by law or public opinion if the operator received, once upon a time, perhaps some forty years ago, his license.

There was a famous German surgeon, Ferdinand Sauerbruch, who ran amok with the scalpel during the last ten years of his life. Everyone around him knew, but, for different reasons—professional, humanitarian, social, personal—all kept silent. This Sauerbruch was not only an eminent surgeon but was also considered an altruist, a saintly, dedicated man, who operated, without ulterior motives, untiringly, day and night, on rich and poor alike. (Beware of dedicated surgeons!) This is an extreme case.[10] But similar maniacs exist around us, and we recognize them. Here we call it "drive" and rather mean it as a compliment.

I personally knew a surgeon whose hands shook and whose gait was less than stable—some kind of paralysis was apparently in progress. In addition, he drank heavily (from after noon). Once I gave anesthesia for an "acute appendicitis" when, drunk and shaking, he successfully went through a right rectus incision but could not locate the appendix. After turning the patient's guts over and over laboriously for twenty minutes, he closed up the patient upon the advice of the general practitioner who assisted him, and called it a day. The patient, miraculously, felt better after this procedure and went home a week or so later. It is worth mentioning that this was a welfare case. No money involved. A pure example of drive: The surgeon could not stop. The doctors at the hospital all knew about his handicap but no one dared, or even wanted, to get involved.

The fact is that there is no way of questioning, limiting, or stopping such activity, provided the patient consents and the surgeon has a license and hospital privileges. In the dressing room young doctors will crack jokes; they know that this particular surgeon opens the chest for any chronic bronchitis or operates for any abdominal pain—but, actually, there is nothing in the contemporary philosophy of surgery that condemns thoracotomy for bronchiectasis or laparotomy on a painful belly due to a pelvic infection.

The surgeons alone, like other narrow specialists, are in no position to establish a different philosophy in their field. The entire medical profession and, of course, enlightened men from other fields should take part in the formulation of a new, sound, realistic philosophy of surgery and medicine. After all, patients—or potential patients—have reason to be concerned about their fate.[11]

X

It is never the medical profession as a whole that evaluates new problems, but always only the narrow circle of specialists in a specific field. To speak about the opinion of doctors in general is, therefore, meaningless. For instance, no other but a cardiac surgeon expresses an opinion on the pros and cons of cardiac surgery, this latest surgical adventure. The cardiac surgeons, of course, feel very optimistic about the future, provided they are given the opportunity to operate ever sooner and more radically. Meanwhile, the fact remains that most cardiac surgery is only a palliation. (And the transplant, at this stage, pure buccaneering.)

An internist, called in for consultation on an elderly, diabetic, arteriosclerotic patient, would never venture an opinion as to the advisability of the operation itself. He will advise as to digitalis or insulin, always assuming that the operation (which in our day usually means a radical operation) "is necessary." Thus an old soul like Robert Frost undergoes radical surgery for malignancy and, a week later, dies from heart failure or coronary occlusion.

In order to perform an abortion, a gynecologist had to seek the opinion and approval of one or two colleagues. It was a good rule. Like any law it often became a mere formality: You do it for me—next time I'll do it for you. Still, it was a step in the right direction, toward an ideal. In a civilized country, is not any other surgery just as important, and the approval and support of one or two fellow physicians should also be sought? Is the removal of a spleen, stomach, uterus, gallbladder a "little nothing" (even if the pathology has been 100 percent established—which is not always the case), and can it be done without further considerations or debates? Is surgery not, after all, an assault on the integrity of body and soul that should be considered as an entity, not as separate units, isolated from each other?

If the opinion and consent of two doctors of different schools of thought were invited in the case of each surgical intervention, the patient himself would also come to know more about his situation, would realize where he stands, and whether he should or should not undergo surgery.

A patient is told that he has an inguinal hernia that should be repaired. The patient has "coverage," which means, as the surgeon puts it, that the operation "will not cost him a penny." Thus, the patient finds himself in a very clear-cut, unequivocal situation. How different it would be if he were informed that he has an inguinal hernia; that some surgeons repair it preventively, even in the absence of clinical symptoms; that some repair only if symptoms appear; that fine, honorable, outstanding physicians belong to either of these schools of thought; and that a repair involves all the risks of a major operation; that it may not turn out a complete success, and can even produce undesirable side effects.

Here is a typical sequence in the patient-surgeon relationship. The patient comes with numerous, vague complaints. After a more-or-less-thorough examination, the surgeon finds a side pathology of which the patient was not aware— hemorrhoids, varicose veins, left lower quadrant pain. He informs the patient that he has hemorrhoids (or varicose veins, or a possible ovarian cyst, or "diverticulitis") and that this particular pathology might very well be the cause of his complaints. "Let's take it out, to start with!" And ahead they go. Months later a major pathology appears, and now it becomes evident that the first, "minor," operation was useless, and most probably harmful.

As the good detective goes after the major suspect, so the doctor must go after the major pathology. And another, even more important consideration: The stress of the unnecessary anesthesia and the crushing trauma of surgery stimulate the growth of a tumor or the formation of metastasis. "To study the influence of anesthetics, tumor suspensions were injected intravenously into 4 groups of 100 rats each...pulmonary metastasis occurred as follows: controls, 37%; pentobarbital, 46%; chloroform, 64%; ether, 55%."[12]

This could mean that the "small" hemorrhoidectomy or saphenous vein ligation has triggered the whole metastatic trend of another pathology that, otherwise, might have been dormant for some years.

Apart from physiological considerations, there are other

dangers in surgery: It is done by men, and men make mistakes; accidents do occur in the operating room. If the common duct of Anthony Eden, then prime minister of England, had not been tied up by a first-class surgeon, the political history of the Middle East might well have been quite different. Cheff Chandler got his aorta ripped while joyfully submitting to a herniated lumbar disk "trifle."

If a patient with intermittent pain in the right upper quadrant is told that he has "gallstones" and that his gallbladder must come out (period!), not much choice is left him. But what if he were told that it could be operated right away or that an attempt at conservative treatment could be made; and that even after the cholecystectomy his pains or discomfort may continue—due to new stones, inflammations, and adhesions; that in some cases a ventral hernia develops as the direct consequence of the operation (as in the case of President Johnson); or a tumor of the vocal cords (due to play-safe intubation—also President Johnson); or an embolism (as in the cases of the late kings of England and Greece); that there is no 100 percent safe play; that every pro has its con and side effect; and that, as long as he is not very miserable and the clinical symptoms are under control and his private and social life not too impaired, it would be wise to postpone surgery (and anesthesia). After such a briefing, the enlightened patient might even go and seek a third advice; this would not be excessive, considering the *irreversibility of major surgery*.

XI

The notion of reversibility and irreversibility is one of the cardinal points of science and of biology in particular. Not much, however, can be found on it in medical literature. And yet, if medicine can be at all defined, it should be defined as the art of reversing the chronic, so-called natural, processes of decline and decay.

Reversibility, we know, is the very essence of anesthesia. Without it the anesthetized body would become a corpse or a vegetative organism. Whatever else anesthesia is, first of all and above all it is reversible. Now, if we were obliged to define surgery in one sentence, we would have to say that, whatever else surgery is, first of all and above all it is irreversible.

Quite a few among the great surgeons of the past were convinced that the insult caused by the scalpel is immense, and overcome only slowly if at all. Therefore, surgery ought to be performed only when absolutely necessary. The "healed" state is achieved by the development of a scar that is here to stay (irreversible). The very opposite of cicatrization is regeneration, which is reversibility par excellence.

Many workers have insisted on the complete anatogonism, in man, between regeneration and cicatrization. "The two phenomena are opposed since cicatrization of the connective tissue blocks regeneration. In various structures, regeneration sets in, but is choked and stopped short by the more vigorous drive of the connective tissue."[13] If the simplest organism is cut in two pieces, each of the pieces will reconstruct the missing part and thus regenerate a complete and perfect entity. The superior species, especially in the mature state, show this characteristic only in an attenuated way; still, the tendency manifests itself. The important fact is that this regeneration—or tendency toward regeneration—expresses itself only if the parts are completely separated or isolated. Should they be brought in contact, as is done in reconstructive surgery, a scar will form, for each part tends to take up in the ensemble only that structure, function, and position proper to that part.

Once again we are reminded that surgery is an adopted child within the medical family. While medicine as a whole is directed toward regeneration and reversibility, surgery, by its very essence, represents an irreversible interference. Sometimes lifesaving, we hasten to add—but always irreversible. This is why it should be performed only if absolutely necessary.

Among the innumerable medical specialities of our time there is one still lacking: that of surgical counselor. He would be a physician with the appropriate training, well-informed in internal medicine and surgery; not in the technique of surgery but in the clinic, prognosis, and postoperative fate. To him the patient could go for advice before deciding on aggressive therapy. The family doctor, busy and too involved, is not fit for such a job and he seldom knows what really goes on in the operating room.

XII

In order to lock up a man in a state hospital, a regular court, with witnesses and experts, must convene. Perhaps a similar, if less spectacular, procedure ought to be instituted for any *elective* hysterectomy or gastrectomy, the final decision resting not with the narrow specialist but with the counselor, the general practitioner and, of course, the patient. (This does *not* apply to emergencies.)

We do not permit people to commit suicide. In England those who attempt suicide are put in jail; here, in a madhouse; in Russia they are sent to labor camps. But in situations having all the characteristic aspects of suicide attempts—under the supervision of a medical specialist!—we do not interfere.

A boy of eighteen or so, who has been suffering a great deal from bad teeth asks the dentist "to take them all out—once and for all" and to fit him with dentures. Can the dentist do it? Yes. Under our civilization he is in the clear. He has the right to pull out all your teeth and fit in a denture, provided you consent—and it matters little whether you are drunk, crazy, or plain stupid. (If he made love to a patient in his office he would be in trouble with the Society, even though the patient consented.)

A girl of sixteen insists on having her nose "fixed"; she gets her parents' consent. As the mother puts it: "She is miserable and drives us mad. We tried analysis but it did not help. . . ." Is this enough for the plastic surgeon to go ahead? Should not the law be able to interfere? After all, New York did legally ban tattooing "for the security of life and health," and what is such cosmetic surgery if not a form of tattooing—or else why could tattooing not be considered "a plastic operation"?

A youngish, good-looking woman with normally developed, well-formed breasts is wheeled into the operating room. Just before anesthesia she frantically hands the nurse an "urgent"

letter to the surgeon in which she implores him to make the
breasts as small as humanly possible. "I hate, I detest, I abhor, I
loathe large breasts . . . and I have to live with my breasts . . . so
please, please. . . ." The letter is accompanied by a photograph
of the Venus of Milo and a hand-drawing by the patient of
Diana's bosom profile, the latter being her ideal. "I am an ama-
zon. . . ." she writes.

Asked after the five-hour-long operation whether his patient
had ever been under psychiatric treatment, the plastic surgeon,
very much surprised, replied: "How should I know?"

A middle-aged woman is admitted for her sixth *major* operation. This is obviously a suicidal manifestation. She has given
her consent, but can such a woman be considered of sane mind?

The peculiar thing about our twenty million plus operations
per year is that they are not at all evenly distributed among our
two hundred million Americans: The bulk have no surgery
whatsoever while the rest have several interventions each. The
rarest species are those who have had only *one* operation
throughout their lifetime.

(It is exactly the same in prisons and penal colonies: one,
first, mistake—then you are sucked in. It would not be surprising to learn that the soaring divorce rate, if broken down,
showed the same built-in mechanism.)

The personal consent of surgical addicts is of no value. Elective surgery should not be performed on the basis of their purely
subjective feelings and desires. Such patients know not what
they are doing; they are psychotics, or they are hypnotized by a
culture that, while indifferent to religion, generates its own, very
primitive, belief in science and technological progress.

The press has come to play a leading part in this general
eulogy of science and her priests. In their constant drive for
something new, the reporters produce every week (or twice a
week) a latest radical operation or an additional wonderful experiment. If, a month later, this "new" radical operation ends in the
death of the patient, or the "new" wonderful experiment turns
out to be a failure, the press, already engaged elsewhere, does
not make an issue of it and in most cases simply neglects to report
on it.

On and off magazines publish autobiographical, illustrated

stories by patients: "How I was cured of cancer." What a good piece of work it would be for an ambitious newspaperman to go and check on those "cured" people, to find out whether they are still around, and in what condition.

The distorted image produced by the press is intended to stimulate further contributions, donations, grants, and the establishment of new foundations that will work along the old, exhausted lines, repeating each other's mistakes and stepping on each other's toes. If we could only stop for a moment and think!

XIII

It is the trend among surgeons to do as many cases as possible. The ego is flattered by the number of patients as well as the money involved. The busy surgeon who runs from case to case, from hospital to hospital, and who hardly has time to see his patients pre- or postoperatively—this busy surgeon makes such an amount of money that after taxes, despite the most judicious advice of his accountant, his dollar is worth fifteen to eighteen cents. And still he is ready to go out at night for an additional (questionable) appendicitis. What drives him? Certainly not the 15 to 20 percent of the dollar. It is obviously something irrational that, like all irrational matters, should be explored, explained, and controlled—especially if other people's bodies and souls are involved. The surgeon's pride is the number of operations he does per annum; this, more than the money earned, is the scale by which he compares himself with his colleagues and competitors.

How far removed we are from the beginning of the surgical era, when the good surgeon was the one who operated the least. If surgery is judgment rather than technique, this judgment should be used in deciding whether to intervene or to abstain; the surgeon who abstains more often than not is becoming a fossilizing species.

There is yet one other aspect to consider: Surgeons, too, grow older, weaker. Their coronary vessels shrink; their sight and hearing deteriorates; their hands begin to shake; their fingers stiffen and their spines play tricks on them after half an hour of bending over the table while trying to "play safe" on their patients.

There is no clear-cut law by which a surgeon, once provided with a license, can be stopped from performing complicated operations. Everybody around him may know that he is not fit, but: It is hard to prove that a man has lost part of his sight or hearing; the field is highly competitive (and we never really approve of other people's work); the ethic code is a peculiar one. To witness against a fellow physician is considered unethical.

In the United Kingdom a fatigue test was performed on pilots. Here are some results: Experienced jet fighter pilots revealed that they were safe for two hours and forty minutes of flying, but not safe after five hours and five minutes without a night's sleep intervening. Three sorties within twenty-four hours they considered safe; more than five unsafe.[14]

Such evaluations by surgeons and anesthesiologists are unknown. And yet it would not hurt to find out the critical point in these professions. One laparotomy? two laparotomies? three laparotomies? Off and on we read about additional tests for car and truck drivers who have reached a certain age. No such suggestions were ever made concerning surgeons. Is this not strange? But to leave such tests in the hands of the parties involved would be like leaving the control of liquor legislation up to the bartenders.

Apart from all philosophical considerations, surgery is also a way of making a living. The economic aspect must therefore be taken into account. As long as the ambitious surgeon has a moral and legal alibi, any conservative trend—which is bound to hit the pocket—is not likely to emerge spontaneously. The only way in which a surgeon is trained to make a living is by operating. And if he does not do it, the fellow on the next block probably will.

Many years ago, when I was still in training, the conviction grew in me that a specialist who charges $350.00 for a cholecystectomy is worth at least the same in cases where he abstains from operating—on condition that he stands behind the patient and is prepared to intervene within the reasonable future.

It all goes back to this case. In a private hospital, a woman in labor presented some difficulties; a cesarian section was contemplated, and a professor of gynecology called in for consultation. He came, examined the patient, and announced: "Leave her alone. She will deliver all right!" After that he stated his fee—an exorbitant one, the same as for a section performed by him.

"To come for half an hour, examine the pelvis, and collect a fortune—what nerve!" was my reaction, and that of a couple of young doctors around.

And yet it was exactly as if he had performed a section—in a lofty, elegant manner. For it so happened that the woman delivered beautifully, without surgery, a few hours later. Incidentally, the professor had left instructions that if the patient did not dilate as anticipated, or if other complications arose, he would be ready to come and perform the section—without additional fee.

To pay the surgeon even if, for the time being, he abstains from operating may well solve many a petit and grand mal of our beloved medicine. The old Chinese approach to the physician's fee was perhaps not so naive!

XIV

It is true that recent advances in anesthesiology, antibiotics, electrolyte balance, etc., have made complicated, exhausting operations on very poor-risk patients possible without *immediate* fatalities. However, this does not excuse the abuses in surgery. Those cancer patients who survive five years and more do so, quite possibly, not because of radical surgery and extensive dissections but despite all this. After all, some patients improve or recover completely with no, or very rudimentary, surgery. Complete cures have been attributed to the reticuloendothelial system and to immunological reactions.

The idea grows that surgery is no answer to cancer. This idea is becoming more and more accepted in serious medical circles. But the philosophy of surgery—and the practice—remains old-fashionedly aggressive. During a span of ten years I once gathered some peculiar statistical data:

1. J. F. Dulles, cancer of colon, died eighteen months after operation;
2. King George V, cancer of lung, died two years after operation;
3. King Paul of Greece, cancer of stomach, died a few days after operation;
4. Robert Frost, tumor of sigmoid, died of heart failure after operation;
5. General McArthur (pathology not clear to me), operated on several times, died three weeks after initial operation.

I do not know of operations on other patients of equally high status. If they were reported in the press, I missed them. An additional list would include: Charles Laughton, Mrs. Robert Wagner, Gary Cooper, Humphrey Bogart, Mrs. George Wallace—all victims of cancer. (However, the fact that they had surgery seems never to have been recorded in the papers.) On the positive side I have noticed only Arthur Godfrey who was operated on for cancer of the lung over five years ago. John Wayne also seems to have made it.

Any newspaper reader can establish his own statistical series and draw the proper conclusions about the value of radical surgery.

Mine is a very small series indeed as compared to the hundreds and even thousands reported by the different medical institutions. However, if the latter are numerically compared to the millions and billions of parameters used in nuclear physics—the one realm where statistical determination has perhaps real value—then it appears that a fair proportion is certainly kept.

Besides, this series has one specific quality: It consists only of people at the very top of the social and economic ladder. These persons were, practically, under constant medical supervision; all the famous checkups were religiously performed. If it were within human power to detect cancer or major pathologies in the earliest stages, it should have been possible in these cases. After diagnosis they were immediately operated upon and the "best" procedures known to science were applied. If early diagnosis, radical surgery, excellent aftercare, were effective, victory should have been theirs.

In this way we arrive at a paradoxical deduction: Given that more than half of major cancer cases die, even under the best possible conditions, three years after the operation, it seems logical that the patient will live the longer, the later he undergoes *radical* surgery. This statement may sound absurd, but it is perhaps permissible to take recourse in exaggeration, considering the formidable position of the modern surgeon that we are challenging.

The fact is that the time has come to initiate the general public into some contradictions of contemporary medicine. It is my conviction that the professional body of physicians is, at the present stage of its activities, simply not able to revise its outdated philosophy without aid from the outside. Physicians have no time for that; not enough general education; no tradition in such wide-reaching elaborations.

Clemenceau, the "father of victory," who during the First World War played a role similar to Churchill's in World War II, used to say: "War is too serious an enterprise to be trusted to the generals." Society has accepted this truth. On top of the military are civilians—elected civilians, in democratic countries. With the advent of nuclear fission there has been a strong trend in the democracies to limit the scientist, the physicist, the professional man, "the man in uniform," in handling directly nuclear weapons and the problems connected with them. This seems a sound idea. The periodically elected officers are the ones to be entrusted with that responsibility. If they need specific information, the experts are at their disposal.

The history of the last fifty years has proven that any insane, pseudoscientific, antihumanitarian, demonic theory or movement can find the support of some world-renowned professor. Salvation may be in the jury: They listen to the contradictory testimonies of different experts and then render the verdict according to their inner conviction.

If war is important, and H-bombs are dangerous, what about health and well-being? Is it not more precious and actual for all of us? Yes, health is too important to be entrusted to the physicians alone.

Part III
MEDICINE
AND THE
SENSE OF WELL-BEING

Medicine is education

I

Primum non nocere. This was the cardinal rule at the time that medicine turned into science. *Primum non nocere.* As a rule of practice, as a goal, and as an ideal. It still is the ideal of internal medicine, far removed from the surgical "play-safe" principle— in fact its opposite. In surgery they tend to open ten bellies for one possible pathology; here, first of all, do no harm—then try to help in whatever way you can. But never harm! That means: Do nothing useless, dangerous, or ambiguous.

Of course, we do prescribe cortisone, poisonous tranquilizers, deadly antibiotics; but no doctor who knows the truth about these wonder drugs rushes to apply them. First he looks for other ways out. Often the practice may be wrong but the ideal is here, firmly established. Yes, the patient comes to the doctor for help but—*primum non nocere.* It may be relatively easy to help in one respect. The question is, how will it affect the rest of the organism? The medical man still thinks about such trifles or, in any case, is supposed to do so.

Some general practitioner may distribute pills: the scored one after meals, the other at bedtime! He sees sixty patients a day, each for five minutes. This is wrong—it is the particular doctor who does wrong (and knows it). The philosophy behind him is still *primum non nocere.* If he adhered to it, he would have to stop his abuses. Here our argument is rather with the cynical practitioner and not, as in surgery, with the idealistic fanatic.

Many improper practices are explained by the fact that the patients ask for them. The doctor comes to see a child with fever: pharyngitis. He prescribes aspirin and forced fluids. Next day the mother complains—no results, how about penicillin? "But there is no indication for penicillin," the general practitioner argues. The mother calls another doctor who gives a shot of penicillin. The following day, the child's temperature is down (which would have happened anyway). The mother is jubilant and the first doctor, the conscientious one, has lost a customer.

57

After several such lessons, he too starts out with routine use of penicillin and other "wonder" drugs.

Again, it is not the philosophy of medicine that is to blame. We must blame the weak doctor, and above all the patient—the latter's mentality, lack of culture, his misunderstanding of what medicine is here for. Unless the patient has a clear idea of what he can and cannot expect from a doctor, no harmony is possible in the patient-doctor relationship. It can never be emphasized enough that modern medicine is possible only in a culturally advanced society.

II

The specialist, when a patient comes to see him, is faced with a rather simple problem: He searches for some familiar abnormality or rather for what, at this stage of our knowledge, seems to us abnormal. Once found, he tries to correct it, even if the patient's complaint was not connected with this pathology.

The internist is the one medical man who must always, by definition, envisage the entire picture that particular patient presents; and in this picture, the general beliefs, the outlook and philosophy of the sick person, play a definite role. In fact, unless the doctor knows how the man plans to use his health, he may not even be able to help him. In short, the philosophy of medicine is connected with the philosophy of life. To save the patient from a bad life and to help him continue to lead a good one—this obviously is within the realm of medicine (Korschinsky).[35] The problem of good and evil is inherent in the medical sciences, for sickness and death are evil and health is good.

"Is the evil only natural insufficiency, imperfection, vanishing by itself with the growth of good or is it a real power by means of temptation governing the universe, so that to overcome it we must have a point of reliance in another order of existence?" It is Saint Augustine who asks this question. According to him, evil has no substance; it is *privatio* or *omissio boni*. Is the same true for illness? Is it *privatio* or *omissio boni*, absence of health and the sense of well-being? Or is sickness a concrete entity in itself, inhabiting and torturing the given organism?

It is not too much to say that even the medicine man, or the magician, already had a philosophy of medicine in accordance with his personal understanding of such and similar life problems. Is old age and illness the loss of a precious, vital gift or, on the contrary, a result of the accumulation of evil, poisonous substances? Different philosophies of medicine have, through the ages, attempted to answer these and similar questions. Should health perhaps be regarded as a system of cosmic laws, reflected in the human organism in such a manner that the free will of the individual naturally coincides with those cosmic laws (every time you hurt yourself, your choice, apparently, went against the cosmic rules)? Or is health rather the end result of a very clever exploitation of the blind forces of nature by a skilful and intelligent operator?

Thus a philosophy may draw on the wisdom of the cosmic powers, instructing the subject to live in harmony with the universal laws that, by definition, are good and God-like. This basically is the natural law in medicine: It considers the universe as friendly toward the living creature, just as Saint Augustine considered every soul born good and Christian. Be this as it may, but to *remain* Christian is certainly exceedingly hard for the soul. And it is just as difficult to protect our sense of well-being on the voyage through the cosmic oceans.

Another, slightly attenuated, moralistic philosophy would consider health as a consequence of a person's general conduct. In a healthy society, the individual who "behaves himself" will always be healthy (and, for that matter, wealthy and wise too). Therefore don't gamble, don't drink, don't. . . .

A complete philosophy may be constructed on the basis of some new observation or a series of such observations that the "discoverer" blows up into a universal panacea. Thus, through history, particular sets of remedies appear and are applied indiscriminately to every patient and every disease. Be it bleeding and leeches, a special diet of mushrooms or yoghurt, extracts of certain plants or glands, tissue therapy, the homeopathic approach or the psychoanalytical—they all have in common that a partially justified remedy is suddenly generalized, sanctified, and made universal.

III

In the 19th century an interplay, an ever-increasing parallelism, between medicine and law developed. Under the influence of progressive ideas the law began to classify many offenders as sick, abnormal, irrational, and, therefore, legally not responsible. Medicine, on the other hand, began to interfere more and more with the private lives and rights of humans. Forced quarantines, vaccinations, sanitation regulations, are all examples of interference in private lives based on medical concepts. "It is against the law to smoke marijuana (or to sniff cocaine)" claims the medical man, or rather the law under the influence of the prevailing medical philosophy. Actually, the restriction of an individual from harming himself could be considered an interference with his constitutional rights. The freedom of the individual to do whatever he pleases with his personal health or to behave as he chooses in case of epidemics or disease has long since become a myth. Health is considered part of the social structure. It is the duty of the citizen to protect his health, in which the state has a vested interest. A member of our society is expected to live healthily and within the law, so as to keep up the accepted way of life and not to interfere with the well-being of others.

As long as the status quo was the rule in all aspects of the state, it could also be maintained as an ideal in medicine. But when all social classes began to move out of their historical nests, creating new opportunities and taking possession of new positions, the status quo broke down along the entire line and there was no way of keeping it up in one isolated area such as national health. There has been an increase in all kinds of pathologies and their variations since the Age of Enlightenment brought a liberation from old institutions, clans, and guilds. Syndromes and pathological units form like species: They mutate and sometimes become extinct.

The afflictions peculiar to the lower classes used to be mutilations and distortions: hunchbacks, dislocations, amputations, ruptures, festering varicose veins, and, finally, TB. Their children suffered from malnutrition, scurvy, rickets, thrush, anemia. The scourge of the middle classes was gout, diabetes, arthritis. The aristocrats suffered from heart diseases, nervous syndromes, brain hemorrhages. (Of course, the periodic classical epidemics were for all who could not travel to a safe place.)

As Proust put it, "Each social class has its own pathology." But with the annihilation of the class barriers, those illnesses did not disappear but overlapped, became universal, all-embracing. Now, in the jet age, even tropical and "racially specific" pathologies are becoming common under our skies.

All this presented the modern medical man with manifold complex tasks and gave him unprecedented authority.

IV

The beginning of the scientific era, in medicine as well as in other fields, was marked by the cause-and-effect dictum. The physical and biological observations accumulating in the laboratories aroused such enthusiasm that all metaphysics seemed to have become worthless. Previously, science had suffered from a confused Church or, rather, from confused church officials; now the entire trend was to get even with religion *on the rational level*—once and for all.

The joke is that the pioneer in the natural sciences, physics, which suffered most grievously from the Church, made such strides that, in our day, it has met with phenomena that *cannot* be explained only in a rational way. Thus the circle is now closed: The snake of rationalism has come to bite its own tail; the philosophy of contemporary physics is becoming no less irrational than the theology of the Council of Trent. With the development of quantum mechanics, new theories appeared and, in order to grasp reality, common sense had to be abandoned. It is as difficult to understand that an electron is a particle and at the same time a wave, and neither a particle nor a wave (and still something else), as it is to rationalize the structure of the Holy Trinity.

But contemporary medicine does not take these latest developments into account. Retarded, materialistic, rooted in obsolete theories, it not only ignores the spiritual plane of human nature but also—and this is most striking—the latest changes in the theories of modern science. The advent of the microscope was a stimulus to the life of medicine. The new revelations of the microscopical *nuclear* universe are still ignored by our medicine.

The empiric, experimental facts accumulated of late in biology and physiology call for a complete revision of the old philosophy of medicine, which is no less naive than the old classical astronomy, than Darwinism, Marxism, and other deterministic theories.

V

This lack of an adequate new philosophy is not confined to medicine. Other fields of our social structure are in the same trouble. The philosophy of law is also retarded and perhaps even in greater danger of fossilization. This must not prevent us from acknowledging that a now-obsolete law may have been of great value and a sign of progress some time ago. But what are we to make of such naive argumentation as this: Because the accused, as a child, saw his mother making love with a stranger, he killed (raped, molested, robbed) a gorgeous blonde—twenty years later? This is an example of how science degenerates into pseudoscience.

The truly great discovery that it is better to let nine criminals go free rather than convict one innocent, now seems questionable. The activity radius has become so wide that the proportions have changed dramatically. Take, for instance, a pharmaceutic manufacturer who is suspected of marketing a dangerous drug. By applying the principle of nine to one, we actually endanger millions of human lives. In such a case it might be better, from the humanitarian point of view, to stop the activities of nine innocent manufacturers than to tolerate one possible criminal.

This legal principle is of special interest to us, since it has its (reversed) counterpart in medicine. "It is better to operate on nine healthy persons than to miss the tenth with the appendicitis." This is the famous play-safe principle. What an alarming contradiction is implied in the claim, on the one hand, that surgery has made tremendous progress, and in the necessity, on the other hand, to open ten bellies to find one pathology!

The sad fact is that the play-safe principle is an illusion. The temptation of safe play has been a persistent one. From antiquity, wise men have warned against it. Among the religious commandments given through the ages, not one orders us to play safe. How did such a shortsighted, materialistic slogan find its way into all aspects of life in the United States, a basically Christian country? Communistic Russia ought to have such a dictum—but they do not. "Play it safe" probably originated in legitimate business and there it might be justified. Transferred to other areas of life, and particularly to life itself (which is an adventure), it does not make sense.

Next to the play-safe principle, it is the question of cause and effect that is the most urgent and the most complicated one to be considered. Causality marked the beginning of the scientific era—the time of entire celestial bodies, organs, systems, and organisms. Since then we have arrived at the atomic, cellular, molecular level, where the cause-and-effect dictum does not hold true. What implications does this have for contemporary biology and medicine? This question needs to be asked at long last.

We are well convinced that bacteria produce substances that interfere with the functioning of the body and can make a person sick. But the body can produce substances that interfere with the functioning of those bacteria. Thus two opposing tendencies are at play. Who wins depends on complex factors, which will perhaps never be fully understood. In any case, it is too simple to call microorganisms the "cause of the disease"; they merely tend to initiate a process that multiple other factors accentuate, change, or neutralize. The same is probably true for cancer: While all research is oriented toward finding a main causal factor, the solution may not be a deterministic one and may lie elsewhere—on the nuclear level, where the principle of indeterminism reigns and freedom of choice is a reality.

The classic example is a two-car collision. If one of the drivers had started out ten seconds earlier (or later), or had stopped to buy cigarettes or slowed down to avoid a squirrel, this particular accident would not have occurred. Again, a slightly different turn of the steering wheel might have changed its character for better or worse. This particular collision was not a predetermined development but, rather, an *accident* that came about by chance. The question of where exactly, when precisely, and how such a collision took place or could have been avoided is unanswerable within our frame of reference.

However, we know for certain that roughly 650 such accidents will occur over next Labor Day weekend in the United States, and we also know that in the course of this year n-thousand breast cancers will show up in this country. We know that a certain percentage will survive five years and more regardless of whether a simple or a radical mastectomy is performed. These cases are statistically predetermined, but *individually*, dynamically, they are free and still have a choice (despite microbes, environment, genetics): They are undetermined.

Life has always been threatened by the terrible forces of nature—by tidal waves, hurricanes, avalanches, earthquakes. But exactly these same forces—and infinitely greater cataclysms—generated our solar system, our planet, our first living cell. Here enters the concept of the *direction* of those currents, winds, explosions, cataclysms: The same element brings death and originates life—depending on the direction.

Something similar may apply to our health. The same forces that create the conditions for abnormal cell mytosis might be used to reverse the process. "A ship can sail with or against the wind; the problem is how to tack" (N. Fedorov).[15] The Normans, who had the art of tacking, conquered all of Europe and reached the Americas. There were at the time courageous warriors among the French, the Italians, the Moslems and the English—but they did not know how to tack. The problem may well be whether the cells of some individuals "know how to tack," avoiding collision with abnormal forces and, after an operation, avoiding metastatic processes (thus surviving five years and more), while the cells of others, egotistical and panicky, begin pulling, each in a different direction, defending only their own interests, destroying each other.

One of the examples of how a deadly wind can be caught in our sails and exploited in our favor is immunization. But here also lies a danger: Exceeding interference with our immunological system may, and should, lead to the general collapse of this system. It is clear that to initiate such danger-fraught interferences requires much more general knowledge and experience than contemporary medical science in its strict sense offers.

Any philosopher, legislator, religious leader is, by the very nature of his occupation, also a physician; for him, too, the people's well-being serves as a beacon. Correspondingly, the doctor who is concerned with the patient's sense of well-being must again become a philosopher, theologian, scientist, even an artist, initiated in the problems of health, harmony, goodness, and freedom. Our medical schools should emphasize the humanities, Greek and Latin texts, for later the student will easily find colleagues to instruct him in how to control diabetes but rarely will come across an individual who will quote St. Augustine or Spinoza.

VI

Instead of starting out on new adventures, modern experimental medicine prefers to repeat, copy, duplicate, spending allotted time and funds on working in the same old direction. The immense amount of doubling and repeating of papers and experiments in our laboratories can be compared only to the process at work in the "best-sellers" of fiction, movies, and musicals.

All research shows the same tendency: toward more aggressive, more radical procedures. After simple mastectomy, radical mastectomy evolved; both proved inadequate and gave poor results. Therefore a new operation was developed in which the entire chest wall is excised. Even preventive amputation of the opposite breast is being recommended now. No one has the imagination to propose a *lesser* procedure—perhaps only excision of the tumor without any far-reaching dissection. The involvement of the lymph glands in cancer has a double meaning: The glands, it is true, are contaminated; but at the same time they represent a last stand, a barrier against the dissemination of cancer cells. By excising this wall of protection, we throw the organism wide open to the invading cells. That explains perhaps the cases of foudroyant propagation of cancer after a thorough dissection. But no one turns around 180 degrees to march in the opposite direction.

How many teams of dogs in how many academic centers and private institutions are bled daily and then given back blood plus oxygen under pressure? Only God knows the extent of this carnage. Every year dozens of "scientific" papers appear on the subject of hemorrhagic shock, all similar to each other; how many more papers are rejected is anybody's guess: The dogs do not speak.

An institution that receives a grant from government or private philanthropy for scientific exploration must spend this amount to be able to apply for new funds. When at a loss for what to do, the easiest way out is to buy dogs—at fifteen or twenty dollars apiece—and bleed them.

From time to time the papers publish arguments for and against vivisection. Some good people claim that vivisection is necessary for humanity; others deny it. Here again the same mistake is made: either-or; yes or no—that is the trap. Is it not possible that all depends on the project by which vivisection is inspired, the purpose for which it is undertaken, and by whom?

We have no clearing house for experiments. Therefore they can be doubled, tripled, endlessly multiplied, not only in the same country and in the same city, but under the very roof of one institution. This is bad—from the humanistic point of view as well as businesswise.

Under the law of the United States, a citizen with a large income can sacrifice any sum, which otherwise would go to the tax collectors, for a scientific research project of his choice. People are usually sentimental: If Mr. N.'s wife suffered from piles (or arthritis) he destines his gift (of the government's money) toward the cure of piles (or arthritis), while in the overall health picture of the country VD or schizophrenia may be in urgent need of research. Others feel obliged to support the fine arts or the opera with their money. Rembrandt's "Aristotle Contemplating the Bust of Homer" was acquired with over four million dollars of such donations that might very well have gone toward the construction of a much-needed new House of Detention for Women. It is obvious that the old house of detention denied everything for which Rembrandt and Picasso stand.

We want to say that in experimental medicine some new planning on the state level is badly needed. There should be a clearing house to establish what is urgent, and what can wait, and what is already being done in several places. There should be some order and a program. Money alone does not make the great society. Grants without a new approach serve only to multiply and copy the old exhausted schemes; people will repeat the same experiments on chick embryos or on the poor dogs for the thousandth time.

Salvation may come from a completely new field. The moon or Mars, while perhaps proving useless for military strategy, may provide an agent to counteract leukemia, or a wide-range genuine antibiotic. This may be called the indirect approach in science. Columbus seeking the western route to India and finding a new continent; Pasteur studying the nature of yeast and discovering a new micro-universe. The indirect approach with a turnabout of 180 degrees. To pour new money in the same direction is like sending more and more soldiers to the same front sector—they only step on each other's toes. Strategy means to create a diversion, a second front.

It is characteristic for our human blindness that most arguments against the space program end with the plea: "Please! There is so much to be done here on earth! Why not rather give those billions of dollars for the fight against cancer?" Who knows but that this very space program will provide an answer in the fight against cancer, and in the meantime our hospitals profit by acquiring, for operating rooms, laboratories, and recovery units, sophisticated electronic equipment—leftovers from the space program.

But it need not be only the moon. Completely new fields of

exploration exist also in our immediate vicinity. Such is one study undertaken in France—the study of death. Not biology but "mortology" or, if you prefer Greek, thanatology. In a documented work on this subject, Hubert Larcher[16] tries to establish the general laws of the postmortem life of the corpse by studying it long after clinical death and by comparing statements of witnesses (many of them doctors) concerning religious specimens that have been preserved through the ages.

His first observation is the tendency toward fluidity. Second, the tendency toward diffusibility of the fluids, with the vascular walls becoming hyperpermeable. If there could be an act of self-preservation and adaptation to the surroundings after functional death—and why not envisage it—these tendencies would be the manifestation of such a phenomenon. The third is the tendency toward homogeneity. Fluids and solids slowly but perfectly mix and become homogenous, sooner or later. Thus, at the end of this physical evolution, the corpse will be bathing in a homogenous mixture imbibing every cell, which during life could have been reached only by means of the cardiovascular system.

From these observations, a possibility of new stages of adaptation and self-defense appears that would make sense only if, somewhere, sometime, a reversibility could be expected to take place.

Is such a body really and completely dead in all possible respects or does it, rather, find itself in another, special form of existence that can perhaps still be reversed?

By saying "nonsense" we do not achieve anything. It is the exploration of so-called nonsense and miracles that makes us scientists. Who among medical doctors, smelling the pleasant fruity odor of a diabetic patient, was not at least once reminded of the old tales about saints who "exuded a sweet perfume"?

VII

Judgment is perhaps the most important quality in a doctor, and an analysis of this quality is, therefore, an important task. One thing is certain; the entire individual expresses himself in his judgment. Everything enters into play—general education, background, special knowledges, skills, creative gifts, convictions, and an interrelation of all main functions such as reason, emotion, intuition, courage, imagination. As Schopenhauer put it: "Of all the intellectual faculties, judgment is the last to mature." (And probably the first to degenerate, it could be added.)

Obviously the narrow specialization of our day tends to impair this wide interplay of all the faculties and cuts off the roots through which our judgment ought to be fed. "Gynecologically (or gastro-enterologically) speaking, this patient should be operated on. Now it is up to you to evaluate him from the general point of view!" Is not such a statement an acknowledgment of the misery of our present-day medicine?

With the accumulation of scientific data it seemed impossible for one man to possess complete medical knowledge, and a trend of specialization and subspecialization set in. It does indeed provide more effective technical possibilities for handling specific problems in more and more limited fields. But the more a physician knows about ears, guts, or bones, the less he is concerned with the general active well-being of the person, even though the textbooks warn him not to fall into this trap. And yet, if we had to define in one sentence what it is that medicine should offer humanity, I would say it is the sense of *general well-being*, physical as well as spiritual, entire, indivisible, full. For health is totalitarian and global in its origins. How can this demand for unity, integration, totality, of an ideal medicine be reconciled with the fragmentation that goes with different specialities?

When an ocean liner approaches the shore and the intricate harbor is already in view, the pilot is brought aboard. Familiar with the reefs, inlets, sandbanks, and currents, only he is entitled to bring in the ship and, later, to guide it out. On the next island or continent, another man will be called aboard to bring the vessel safely into the haven.

But there always remains the question of the great, the majestic, navigation on the seven seas, and this responsibility lies with the captain. No native pilot, experienced and qualified as he may be, can replace those navigators who think in terms of the vast, mysterious oceans. The entire philosophy of these two species of man is different; different their backgrounds, education, methods and attitudes, aims and ideals.

If the specialist, like a pilot, navigates with authority the channel between middle and inner ear or between anus and sigmoid or between vulva and ovaries, then the internist ought to be—and originally was—that great captain of the seven seas, navigating on the physiological ocean, making use of the winds even when they oppose him, leading the vessel and its cargo safely across. But in this case, the captain must know the destination, the currents, and the character and value of the cargo; he must know the purpose of the voyage. This physician-captain requires not only an education in medicine, physiology, psychology, but also a philosophical approach to the human condition. The doctor must again become what he used to be—a philosopher, a wise man, a teacher of life. For if the patient wants the physician to prolong his life—*ad infinitum* if possible—then the physician must also be able to instruct the patient how to live, after he has been cured, so as to preserve his restored health. To be able to give such instruction, a vision and the knowledge of essential basic values are needed, as well as the courage and will to apply them. This, however, is precisely what our culture opposes. Even if a doctor has beliefs and convictions—and most of them do—he will not express them in his office. It would be considered unethical and never good for business.

In the past, where an integral faith existed, a corresponding philosophy of life was possible; the wise man, the priest, the physician, raised their voices in matters of general conduct and the pitfalls of daily existence. Not that this is not done today. It is done, but under altogether different assumptions. The main criterion is utility, comfort. The notion of good and evil is ignored. And yet, good and evil may be a universal reality, and the lack of adequate signals may become a source of confusion and chaos on the cellular and autonomous level.

Instead of feverishly looking for a new speciality, the general practitioner should recognize this natural need: It is not enough to tell the patient "take it easy and relax." There is much more to it. To envisage all the evils of tension, passions, and competition; to know how to transform and neutralize them from the start—and to teach all this—requires an entire new discipline and culture.

We tell the patient that smoking is bad for him and that he ought to stop it. Such advice is of no value. The doctor should know how to instruct the patient in such and similar tasks, should be able to help him "help himself"—and for this the doctor too ought perhaps to be able to give up smoking. This would give him a specific inner experience and also the moral authority to influence the patient.

A rather famous professor of philosophy was strongly advised to give up cigarettes. His life became hell; he hid in closets to take a few illegal drags. His wife told him once: "I could not care less about a philosopher who recognizes an evil but cannot overcome it!" Here, in a nutshell, is the pathetic difference between the sage and a professor of philosophy. We have enough teachers of different subjects and masters of different techniques, but we lack the sage—there seems to be no room for him. (The Eastern, so-called backward, countries have exactly the opposite problem.)

An even more impressive example is the case of Freud. In 1923 Freud, a heavy smoker, became aware of a lesion in his mouth. Surgery was performed. In the years to come, Freud experienced repeated formation of new leukoplakias and precancerous lesions that were treated surgically more than thirty times. Finally a new malignancy manifested itself. Dr. Schur, Freud's physician and biographer, reports: "I enquired about his habits and could not avoid discussing his smoking. I soon recognized that this was one area where Freud had not established the "dominance of the ego." After periods of anginal pain he might give it up for some time, but soon he would greet me with a disarming and touching gesture—"Well, I've started again!"[17] All the psychoanalysis through which Freud passed did not help him to free himself from such slavery.

VIII

If the personality is split, if our culture is split and full of contradictions, Christian churches multiplying, political parties, nations, governments, burgeoning, then it is only natural to have a broken, fragmented medical science, aimed not at the integral living person but at his different organs and parts, which are regulated by antagonistic systems. A new medicine can appear only after an integration of all other aspects of our cultural life. Meanwhile we must do our best in a divided world.

When the American workers began to organize, the leaders had the choice between vertical and horizontal partition. They chose the latter. Thus into the same union enter several different branches of industry that only indirectly belong to the same group. Such classification created a great deal of confusion in the beginning, but has apparently paid off in the long run. The same could have been done with medical specialization to everyone's advantage.

An obstetrician routinely delivers hundreds of babies, the greater part of whom could have come into this world with the help of a midwife or, for that matter, of a policeman or any kind-hearted neighbor. The obstetrician has to call in a pediatrician to take care of the infant. This pediatrician, in his turn, runs from one child to another, scrutinizing inflamed tonsils that any general practitioner or even any qualified registered nurse could diagnose and treat successfully with aspirin. And yet, those pediatricians are highly trained in infectious diseases, can perform difficult spinal taps, and make the differential diagnosis of obscure forms of polio or encephalitis, regardless of whether they occur in infants or adults. But here again it is against the rules of the board of specialities to call a pediatrician for a middle-aged man with symptoms of meningitis.

Notice that in England 75 percent of all deliveries are done by *student* midwives and that the survival rate is better than in the United States where all deliveries, at least in principle, are performed by medical men. In Russia, a gigantic corps of nurse attendants and medical aides takes care of most of the routine cases, apparently with success.

In every speciality there is about 75 percent of routine work that could be delegated to technicians without ill effects. On the other hand, all specialities overlap, so that the same man may be considered competent in two or three adjacent fields. Thus the bread and butter of ophthalmology is refraction, which any intelligent technician could be trained to handle in most cases. This would save 75 percent of the ophthalmologist's time, which he could then use to peep into ear, nose, and throat, or perhaps for neurosurgery (why not?).

A highly trained anesthesiologist uses no more than six or seven drugs, tubes the patient endotracheally, and routinely sticks a needle into the spine. Some of these procedures are done as well by technician nurses; but in order to digitalize the patient or read his EKG or bronchoscope him—the latter a procedure very similar to intubation—the anesthesiologist must, for legal reasons, call in an internist or an ENT man. Considering that an anesthesiologist is a full-fledged medical doctor with training in general medicine before the residency, this does not make sense.

Should an internist not be willing and able to diagnose an abdominal surgical pathology without relying on the surgeon? Nowadays, an internist who examines a patient with the well-known symptoms of acute peritonitis (pain, rebound, rigidity) simply calls it a "surgical belly" and refers the patient to a surgeon who, naturally, advises immediate radical operation.

A tragic farce takes place at the sickbed. Two competent physicians deliberate about the fate of the patient. Their jurisdictions are sharply divided. It seems improper for them to overlap. And thus it happens that, in the region where their two fields touch, the patient is actually not covered. This is how it comes about that men like McArthur and Frost are operated on—with deplorable results.

All myocardial infarcts are the result of "trauma," be it mechanical, biochemical, or metabolic (the slowdown of coronary circulation also acts as a trauma to the myocardium). By hurting the heart, directly or through the ribs, a fatal accident can be caused. Yet we constantly massage the heart, break ribs, rupture the cardia, apply direct force for long periods of time, and then hit the heart with an electric shock—all this as "emergency medicine," in order to restore the cardiac beat to normal. It is hardly possible to imagine a more paradoxical and nonsensical procedure. And even more paradoxical is the fact that the internist, who in his office would not let anyone touch the chest-wall of a middle-aged patient with the slightest degree of force, consents to such procedures, as long as they occur outside his jurisdiction (in the OR).

The Russians, who started emergency resuscitation, transfuse blood under pressure into the radial artery: circulating in reverse toward the aortic arch, the blood exercises a kind of gentle massage that does no harm and can, perhaps, achieve some good.

Of course, a young person whose heart rate has slowed down for a second after an accident may be helped by a momentary, direct or indirect push upon his thorax. But "massages" lasting forty minutes on elderly chronic cardiac patients serve only to traumatize or even rupture the heart; at least this is what usually happens. The internists know, and keep silent, while surgeons and anesthesiologists think up ever more prolonged, complicated, and traumatizing forms of massage to "restore the life" of the patient for a day or a week.

Recently a great debate took place concerning the use of anticoagulants in coronary patients. The opinions were divided—which proves only that both schools of thought are still in the dark. However, it was interesting to note that most cardiologists took a stand for the continuous use of anticoagulants; the opposition came from internists. Here again, the specialist—in this case the cardiologist—was, like the pilot, concerned only with bringing the ship out of the bay, while the internist thought in terms of the entire voyage on the open ocean. (The reef to avoid, here, is possible general or brain hemorrhage, such as Richard Nixon's post-operative collapse.)

IX

During the process of restoring and healing the organism, two aspects must always be kept in mind: (1) The natural tendency of the organism toward restoration and cure; and (2) the interference from outside for the same purpose.

These two processes more often than not hamper each other. In infectious diseases, the introduction of chemicals and antibiotics tends to kill the microorganisms but, at the same time, attacks the cells of the organism; in X-ray treatment, we expose cancer cells to deadly rays but, at the same time, cause normal cells to be destroyed and also hamper the natural, immunological processes.

The problem in therapy is how to destroy harmful agents without sacrificing normal tissue and the natural trend of self-defense that, in some cases, may be the most important factor. We said already that the microorganisms do not *cause* the disease; depending on their "attitude" (their general state), the cells of the organism may accept or reject the infection.

The interrelation of therapeutic agent and self-defense mechanism is the eternal paradox of medicine which, by implication, can never be completely resolved. This could be expressed in a formula similar to Heisenberg's: $dP \cdot dQ = H$; P is the therapeutical Potency—physical, chemical, biological, whatever; Q is the natural, restoring Quality of the organism; H is the *constant* that no improvement of technique can change (like Planck's h).

By improving or increasing P, Q accordingly diminishes— and vice versa. Their multiple is constant. You cannot go beyond this H (as in quantum mechanics). In radical surgery followed by X-ray treatment, the therapeutic part approaches the maximum, so that little is left for the inner immunological processes. What one of the great surgeons said—"I applied the dressing and God cured him"—is here no longer applicable. We try to do everything, without leaving an opening for God or nature. We play it safe! The few spontaneous cures of cancer known to literature are attributed to the reticuloendothelial system, which can so easily be destroyed by drastic interferences.

In addition to the direct interference with the immunological processes, all therapeutic agents and, of course, surgical interventions produce side effects. Side effects are considered "a nuisance" in the tacit hope that, some fine day, they will vanish altogether. Such hopes are unjustified. Side effects are an inner necessity, expressed indirectly through $dP \cdot dQ = H$ (which conveys the relationship between Potency of "drug" and restoring Quality of the organism). It is clear that no progress in pharmaceutics or in technique can do away with those side effects. As in Heisenberg's indetermination principle, the improvement of our tools and technique will not change the universal constant (as long as we think in terms of cells, molecules, and atoms). Of course, all doctors know about side effects; but that they can never be eliminated, *by definition*, seems to arise from modern quantum physics.

The number of "wonder drugs" is rising steadily and the amount and danger of side effects grows in geometrical proportion—for these drugs increasingly weaken the self-defense mechanism. Allergies and shock due to antibiotics and serums; electrolyte imbalance due to new diuretics; new infections caused by previously harmless microorganisms; psychosomatic syndromes after specific treatments; women harmed due to anti-baby pills; babies born crippled due to the mother's addiction to "harmless" drugs. All these are side effects. And so are blood discresias, blindness, endocrinian imbalance, peptic ulcers, collagene diseases. In addition, our tests also expose the patient and do harm.

Some workers evaluate the percentage of iatrogenic complications as 20 percent, without taking into account that iatrogenic effects occur in every treatment, even if they do not manifest themselves obviously and directly.

Side effects are just as numerous in surgery: adhesions, prolapses, ventral hernias, causalgias, impaired circulation, even phantom pain, are side effects. Very often a sequence of operations follows a chain of side effects, eliminating (or trying to eliminate) each one in the order in which it was produced.

And one more thing: The patient adapts to his pathology; he makes a complementary effort (Selye's theory of general adaptation syndrome evolves along these lines). When the pathology is removed or displaced by surgery, the old adjustment becomes a source of new pathology. A patient with a displaced vertebral disk curves his spine in such a manner as to protect himself from pain and injury. After removal of the pathological disk, the patient's compensatory effort becomes a nuisance and calls for new adaptation or new intervention.

The physician acknowledges all this but states: "I prescribe a dangerous drug or procedure only if the patient would be much worse off without it. This is a calculated risk!"

A "calculated" risk would imply consideration of all the elements involved. But to be able to grasp all these elements, the doctor must be more than a specialist. His knowledge must extend to the whole of human life, physical as well as intellectual and spiritual. It may be that one element ignored can make the entire "calculation" false. And more often than not it is false.

In law, too, the indetermination formula finds its expression. The task of the Constitution is to protect society without interfering with the rights of the individual. However, this ideal is not obtainable. In accordance with $dP \cdot dQ = H$ we always either infringe upon the Privacy of the individual or destroy the Quality of society, since H is a constant.

X

The formula $dP \cdot dQ = H$ suggests three possible philosophies of medicine that, under different disguises, have manifested themselves through the ages. One of these tends toward radical, determined, aggressive interference, relying on exogenous, artificial means. This philosophy, which we might call the Surgical, is now at its peak and has taken over all aspects of medicine. For what else is the prescription of massive doses of cortisone—usually in diseases with unknown etiology—whose action is obscure and whose side effects are numerous and dangerous, if not a manifestation of this philosophy? What else is the administration of massive doses of X-ray? What is electroshock treatment?

The second philosophy is passive, leaving the main work to the salutary natural processes of the organism, supporting gently, here and there. The credo of this school might be defined by the saying that "the difference between a good doctor and a bad one is enormous, but there is hardly any difference between a good doctor and no doctor at all."

But there is a third approach: The natural processes of self-defense must be elicited, provoked. The salutary, restoring, immunological response is stimulated. An illustration of this philosophy is the modern trend toward multiple repeated immunizations. However, quantity and variety of the agents play a role. There are limits for memory, and an optimal time to learn a subject. Chaotic overloading via vaccinations may lead to a general *immunological collapse*. Recent studies have shown that measles vaccine blocks smallpox immunity. An inhibitor, "interferon," was found in many other experiments. (The result of intensive immunization included "an abnormal serum protein electrophoretic pattern, elevated serum hexosamines, a high incidence of lymphocytosis, unexplained abnormalities of renal function and liver function, and a high incidence of serum antigammaglobuline activity."[18]) It should be mentioned here that cancer metastases are triggered by smallpox vaccination. Any interference with the immunological system of cancerous patients is madness—and surgical trauma, too, is an interference. The Asian flus and the winterly saturnalias of immunization against viruses started some years ago. It was at about that time that the United States went through the famous massive immunization against polio; could there perhaps be a connection?

It would be a mistake to consider the self-defense mechanism of the individual as an ideally positive protective system. What could be more of a blessing than a heart transplant? A man with a diseased, collapsing heart is offered in exchange the normal organ of someone else who cannot use it any longer! The operation, technically speaking, has been a complete success. No direct complications ensue. But soon, too soon perhaps to warrant the tremendous "investments," the patient with the transplant dies. He dies because he *rejects* this salutary organ as a foreign body, rejects it due to his omnipotent, blind self-defense mechanism. To put it succinctly if paradoxically: He dies because of his stubborn instinct for survival.

After a certain point the self-defense mechanism begins to defeat its own purpose. The famous spasm of the larynx, elicited when a foreign body approaches or only seems to approach it, may lead to cardiac arrest and death. A drowning man may choke to death the friend who swam out to help him—and often both go down to the bottom. A bleeding man constricts his vascular system to such a degree that brain and kidneys are completely cut off from circulation (and irreversible damage occurs). Another often-fatal kind of self-defense is the increase of coagulability of the blood under stress—also meant as self-defense and often resulting in the production of emboli. The patient on the operating table who fights the anesthesia from induction to the very end—on all levels with different means—also does it for self-preservation and thus may come close to disaster.

Several years ago a huge lake was to be artificially created somewhere in Africa. Before flooding the territory, officials and volunteers went over it in an attempt to save as much of the wildlife as possible. A large number of animals were indeed rescued and transported to new habitats. But the "strongest" put up a resistance; they fought and escaped salvation. It was practically impossible to help them. In this case, we might say, it was *not* the fittest who survived. In short, self-defense of an organism is good only up to a point, beyond which the blessing becomes an evil. (Perhaps $dP \cdot dQ = H$ applies here too, with the self-defense mechanism to be considered as an agent acquired, previously, from without?)

The diseases resulting from Selye's general adaptation syndrome are also expressions of an irrational exaggeration of the self-defense mechanism. In many instances the pathology resulting from adaptation is greater than the inconvenience that triggered the adaptation. This happens in oversensitive, mixed-up, trigger-happy specimens. What else is psychosis if not a product of the self-defense mechanism that, at great cost, "saves" the organism from some, often small, danger or insult?

XI

Our civilization is based on an erroneous concept of adaptation and adjustment. "Well-adapted, not-so-well-adapted, maladjusted," this is the leitmotiv of psychiatry, education, social science. How many generations of adolescents will be deformed and invalidated thanks to these pseudoscientific assumptions?

Should we adapt ourselves so easily and eagerly? Ought we really to adjust, swing with the tide, join them (if we cannot lick them)? Does it not mean to give priority to the immediate, small profit over the great commitment, the only valuable one in the long run?

Herman Melville, in Moby Dick: "How wonderful is it then—except after explanation—that this great monster, to whom corporeal warmth is as indispensable as it is to man; how wonderful that he should be found at home, immersed to his lips for life in those Arctic waters! where, when seamen fall overboard they are sometimes found, months afterwards, perpendicularly frozen into the hearts of fields of ice, as a fly is found glued in amber. But more surprising is it to know, as has been proved by experiment, that the blood of a Polar whale is warmer than that of a Borneo Negro in summer.

"It does seem to me, that herein we see the rare virtue of a strong individuality, and the rare virtue of thick walls, and the rare virtue of interior spaciousness. Oh, man! admire and model thyself after the whale! Do thou, too, remain warm among ice. Do thou too live in this world without being of it. Be cool at the equator; keep thy blood fluid at the Pole. Like the great dome of St. Peter's and like the great whale, retain, O man! in all seasons a temperature of thine own."

It is not the first nor is it the last time that a poetical or religious vision corrects pseudoscientific reasoning. To adjust, to adapt, to compromise so eagerly, violently, blindly, is perhaps the shortest way to extinction.

According to modern genetics, all vital experiences are passed on to the genes under the label of "information"; the cells honestly transmit this information, from generation to generation, through ages and eons; in fact, organic life is conserved and evolves due to this "memory" on the cellular level.

This essentially deterministic theory can no longer be supported without taking into account freedom of choice on the nuclear level. But suppose that, at least for a given time, it *were* true. May we then ask a simple question: Of what practical use to me is an information that was acquired by my cells when they dwelled in the stages of a sponge, a fish, an amphibian or a monkey? Is this old information, far from being an asset, not rather a liability, a nuisance, a dangerous handicap? Should I not, if I had any sense, try to rid myself of this kind of information, lest I choke at the first occasion on a crumb of bread, suffer cardiac arrest before I reach the shore, refuse help that is honestly offered me and pull the friend, who swims out to save me, down to the bottom of the sea?

Recently a study was conducted that, apart from its practical implications, sheds new light on the contradictions of self-defense. It concerned patients with malignant melanoma. The technique consisted in matching two patients with the same type of malignancy and implanting in the thigh of each an excised piece of the other's tumor. The implant, of course, was rejected. But now the white cells of each patient caused regression and even disappearance of the pathology when transfused into the other patient.[19] The theory behind this may be that, unable to protect themselves directly, they succeeded in the act of self-defense only after helping their neighbor.

Under the changed conditions of our civilization, our archaic, overly egotistic mechanism of self-defense has become an obsolete apparatus. An ameba is educated to devour all the nutritive cells that come its way; but if and when cells of our organism begin to devour neighboring tissues, cancer ensues. If our cells had any sense they would free themselves from that useless "'amebian" information. It is quite possible that they are indeed doing precisely that! In reproducing themselves, they try to wipe out obsolete information and reverse to a previous state, a state of innocence. There is no reason to consider one theory—the theory of genes meticulously coding all information of previous experiences—as highly scientific, and the other—of genes trying to rid themselves of useless, outdated information—as speculation or "metaphysics."

Our autonomous system of course takes part in all such processes. But, by violently and blindly pulling all its strings, we often confuse the cells and throw them off balance (especially since they consist of numerous mini-cells, all with their own "proto-memories"). Thus they finally make a fatal mistake, give up some *vital* information—and chaos and pathology ensue. If medicine were what it was meant to be, we would teach the patient not to defend himself in such a violent, blind way. A little defense and adaptation may be good; a lot is suicidal! This brings us to the problems of the autonomous system.

XII

The most serious, responsible processes of the human organism are performed by the involuntary (autonomous) system. It is as if nature did not trust just any taxpayer with the responsibility for a conscious control of his most important functions, such as cardiovascular performance, glandular secretions, biochemical changes, peristalsis, and, above all, the interplay of all those and other actions. However, it is a myth that these are altogether involuntary processes that cannot be influenced.

In the East, in the so-called backward countries, there has been from the times of antiquity a definite accumulation of knowledge concerning the control of the autonomic or vegetative system. The stories of yogis buried alive or walking barefoot through burning embers, seemingly enjoying it, are perhaps slightly exaggerated. But many witnesses (medical authorities among them) have watched those naked gentlemen come to the river and, sitting down in it, suck water into the colon through the rectum, thus reversing the normal direction of the peristalsis. Every morning, for hygienic reasons, these people depend on this peculiar enema, which may very well be more important than the brushing of one's teeth. The peoples of the West, highly developed and civilized, have in the course of their tremendous technical progress lost all vestiges of such knowledge which, in fact, is neither esoteric nor miraculous. When we feel uncomfortable, we pay the doctor and get a laxative or radical surgery. As Tacitus puts it in the *Annals*: "The Emperor Tiberius always made fun of doctors and of those who, having been alive for thirty years, still did not know what was good and what was bad for their organism and had to seek advice from strangers."

The story of Alexander the Great, who cut the Gordian knot thus "liberating" the wise man from his tedious task and saving him much time (for time is money), is often told in our schools to general approval and satisfaction. And yet, the point of the story is always missed.

The disentangling of a knot was a spiritual chore and part of the basic training of the East. Monks, bonzes, future leaders, and kings worked for months or even several years on one or several knots; while fingering the·rope they continually meditated, so that, at the end of the process, it was not only the rope that had been untangled but something in themselves had also become straightened out and many personal problems solved (without psychiatrists). In our civilization, the remnant of all those knots is the rosary: pious men say their prayers while fingering it and thus arrive at inner peace. (Knitting women also experience the same.)

Now that great barbarian who spoke Greek but who was really Macedonian, Alexander, son of God and/or Philip, came upon this emaciated prince who was struggling with an enormous knot and naively thought that the problem consisted really and solely in undoing it. Of course the superficial aspect of the puzzle is readily solved with the sword (or scalpel). He struck the knot with his weapon—basically achieving nothing. His soldiers and generals applauded, and so do we. The look of contempt the natives around cast at Alexander was neither noticed nor described.

XIII

Most chronic diseases are due to a disturbance of the autonomic nervous system. A stomach ulcer, for instance, results from hypersecretion of gastric juice, which causes irritation and spasms. The surgeon steps in and, if lucky, eliminates the anatomical lesion (without however straightening out the systemic distortion), once again proving the palliative nature of surgery. Basically it is a symptomatic approach, and palliatives or symptomatic treatments are the lowest point of medicine.

Immense technical progress has been achieved by Western civilization but in the process important knowledge has been lost; many fields have become ignored and some capacities completely neglected. Direct influence of the individual upon his own autonomic nervous system and sense of well-being is never considered, while actually there is no reason for neglecting this aspect of another great culture.

We all remember from our childhood how, after having eaten too many apples or plums, we were suddenly gripped by intestinal colics. Desperately fighting the acute urge we would run to the toilet. Just at the moment when we had reached it and had lowered our pants, the extreme need would become unbearable. If the bathroom was close by, that moment arrived sooner; if it was farther, we subdued our urge that much longer. Is this not an example of control of the involuntary system?

During the last decades that were so rich in war and disaster, we had reports about pilots who, wounded and in agony, accomplished their missions, landed their planes safely, and only then collapsed. And, of course, there is the famous story about the young aide-de-camp who galloped across the battlefield with a report for Napoleon. "But you are wounded," the Emperor said, noticing blood on the young man's uniform. "No, Sire, I am killed," answered the youth and fell lifeless from his horse.

Any cardiologist knows that most coronaries occur on weekends or during vacations; not when the patient is occupied, creative, active, but after he has accomplished his duty and is "relaxing."

This peculiarity of humans, to stretch their efforts to the utmost and to extend their lives in order to accomplish what they consider important, is a well-documented phenomenon. What if the important "mission" were to be stretched further, and still a little further? What if every agonizing, so-called common man had a great aim in life and refused to die before having reached it? What if he, his entire person, in harmony with each cell, knew such a goal and cultivated it?

Control of the involuntary activities offers tremendous possibilities, and nothing in our civilization collides with this idea except our constant lack of time. On the other hand, leisure time is increasing—the problem is how to use it adequately. Time is the most important therapist and teacher. It takes years of wrongdoing (active or passive) to develop a chronic pathology—and it must take years to cure it. There are no shortcuts in biology. We may learn how to grow chickens faster and larger; but the taste will be affected—it is no longer a real chicken. The same goes for fruit and vegetables. You can read books faster and faster, and even in the form of digests of digests, but that which appears from one page of the original text of a great writer, read and reread slowly and repeatedly, will be missed.

A doctor inquires about his patient's hobby. Told that it is fishing, he advises the patient to take a vacation and do a lot of fishing. The patient, probably, has no business fishing. In our civilization, where most jobs are meaningless, tasteless and exhausting (only good to "make a living"), the so-called hobby ought to be highly significant, serious, complex, to help the man fulfill himself. In fact, it could become a way of making a living. A bi-professional way of life goes with other duplications of contemporary society: bilingual, bifocal, bi-familial. The amount of emigration all over the world makes us bi-national (or multinational) as well.

A society of bi-professional or multi-professional individuals seems the order of the day. A doctor can enjoy his profession and be good at it only if he sees about ten patients a day; fifty consultations daily make for a miserable way of life. The same for the barber, the lawyer, the electrician, the art critic. Why not combine two professions? It would only be a question of proper organization. Soil, too, gets exhausted, and we sow clover after corn, then potatoes, and then corn again, in order to get the best possible crop.

The question of fulfillment and well-being is of primary importance for the person, indeed for each single cell. When a gland, meant to secrete, is blocked and cannot eject its product, abcesses form and irreversible pathology follows. The sense of well-being is complex and not easily defined. It seems to depend on an interplay of various systems, organs, perhaps cells, all of them in a happy harmonious state. This ideal state may exist under the obvious, abundant (objective) conditions of youth and love and holidays, of satisfaction from career or athletic achievements, but it can also come into being—for no apparent reason—in a winter season full of sneezing and rain, in some middle-aged, not too healthy person. This is the important part: There need not be an apparent reason for it. This sensation does not seem causally determined. It comes from inner sources of the organism (or from the cosmos) and speaks to us without words. It is irrational, intimately conceived, and should be considered the expression of an achieved harmony.

Strangely enough, the sense of well-being is nowhere discussed in textbooks or encyclopedias of medical science, although it is sometimes mentioned as a state characteristic of the organism when recuperating from some danger or disease (mainly convalescence after infectious diseases of childhood).

It is a sign of wisdom, maturity, and good intentions that the patient seeks this feeling of well-being. The mistakes come when he seeks it at all costs and by all means and for himself alone. There is a possibility that people cannot achieve a state of well-being exclusively for themselves. This manifests itself—to a greater or lesser degree—in all of us, and throughout history many have found their sense of well-being by taking care of their neighbor. (If you hit your offender, it is a purely egotistic, materialistic situation, without long-lasting joy or satisfaction; but if you knock down the offender of your neighbor, it may become a highly spiritual and idealistic act.)

There is a reality of the lost paradise in the interrelation and happy interplay of all members of a community (comparable to the happiness experienced by a harmoniously functioning organism). Thus, in the long run, the sensation of well-being is as impossible in a society where some are suffering as it is out of the question in an individual whose organs and cells are under special stress or pain.

The patient remembers this sense of well-being (from his childhood or perhaps even earlier times) and wants to go back to the lost paradise. Reversibility, reversibility, reversibility—the inner cry of all sufferers. Back to youth, strength, happiness; back to the lost horizons, lost friends, lost possibilities.

But here comes the old-fashioned pseudoscientist and tells the patient: "Be reasonable. Be mature. The thermodynamic processes are irreversible. Be strong and kill, as long as you are able to; when you weaken, the fittest will do the same to you. Take these pills twice a day. Relax and submit to the laws of science!" The patient swallows the pill. But can one wonder that he is not satisfied even if his pain is relieved?

In a society where everyone is stuffed with tranquilizers, barbiturates, or narcotics, the natural sense of well-being must gradually change and vanish, to be replaced by a prefabricated, artificial comfort.

XIV

One of the great questions concerning health and the sense of well-being is whether health is a relationship of all the multiple units of which the organism consists, a harmony of all cells and parts, or something absolute, like ideas or forms of beauty and truth. Is beauty a relationship of parts that can be measured and explained or is it an abstract, preexisting phenomenon, independent of us?

How often does a specimen of grace and beauty fail to stand up to rational analysis? Similarly, how often does a medical examination uncover some pathology, while the patient himself manifests a sense of well-being and seems happier and healthier than others who, at the moment, do not present pathologies or abnormalities but who "do not feel like living"? Is all this of some objective value? Is the loss of the sense of well-being perhaps due to several pathologies (their interplay) and not to a single one that remains isolated? Whatever it may be, we repeat: An ideal medicine should keep this general well-being in mind, and lead the patient back to it.

What else does the patient seek when he or she arrives at the doctor's office? Does he need encouragement and palliations? It is the state of well-being the patient wants restored, a state that everyone, presumably, has experienced at some time in his life.

To reverse the process! This universal longing finds its expression in all main aspects of our culture. Art seeks the same results—by other means. What is Proust's "Remembrance of Things Past" (or, as it should rather be called, "The Search for Time Lost") if not an attempt to restore and reverse? For time is perhaps lost because it was not used properly. What is Tolstoi's *Childhood*, wherein he exclaims: "Happy, happy childhood, that blissful time never to be recalled! How can I help loving it and cherishing its bright memories? Those memories refresh and elevate my soul, they are a source of never-ending joy to me. . . ." What is this if not an attempt, by verbal magic, to recreate the past?

And here is Thomas Wolfe in *Of Time and the River*: "For now the child or someone in the house was speaking, calling to him; he heard great footsteps, soft but thunderous, imminent, yet immensely far, a voice well-known, never heard before. He called to it, and then it seemed to answer him; he called to it with faith and joy to give him rescue, strength, and life, and it answered him and told him that all the error, the old age, pain and grief of life was nothing but an evil dream; that he who had been lost was found again, that his youth would be restored to him and then he would never die, and that he would find again the path he had not taken long ago in a dark wood." That same path Robert Frost evokes:

> I shall be telling this with a sigh
> Somewhere ages and ages hence:
> Two roads diverged in a wood, and I—
> I took the one less traveled by,
> And that has made all the difference.

In the art of painting, the portrait is a decisive attempt to "freeze" the person in a state of perfection (or perhaps to bring the subject back to this state and freeze it there).

The concepts of appeal and amnesty are the highlights of civilized jurisprudence.

Ask your butcher or the grocer, listen to exclamations in the supermarket, and you will hear: "If only I could bring back my youth, if only I could feel, act, think, eat, drink, as in my youth!"

The overwhelming, permanent attraction of gambling is still another expression of the same force: With each new deal of the cards or start in the races, a new beginning in life is made possible. Reversibility! (Such vulgar manifestations, too, are of great significance.)

The supreme tendency of every organism, system, cell, consciously or subconsciously, to reverse to a previous perfect state and to start all over again, which manifests itself regardless of time and place—on the mountains, in big cities, subterraneously and on the prairies, by day and by night—this supreme urge is as universal as the force of gravitation, and must find some concrete and constant projection on our being, at least on the cellular level.

Religion in its turn points toward resurrection, immortality, and a familiar paradise (or reincarnation). Reversibility is not negation of time; it is change of order, it is a transfiguration of time. So are poetry and music, where one sequence achieves perfection and thus sticks out of historical times, becomes eschatological.

As for science—does it not seek control over the entire four-dimensional continuum that, of course, includes time?

Thus medicine, philosophy, science, religion, art, all supreme human functions, are storming the same walls—with different means. If I had to answer the short question "What is culture?" in one sentence, I would say: "Culture is defined by the body of reversible processes known to a given society."

It is clear that in a closed society the transfer from one social stratum to another, even from one profession (guild, union) to another, is difficult or impossible; irreversible. The same goes for religious, ethnic, psychological barriers in a primitive society. In some countries a person cannot possibly change his name—or has to go through hell to achieve it.

In the ideal society, not only the underprivileged, the colored, the derelict, will attain all opportunities and privileges, but also the old, sick, ugly, and handicapped. They shall be enabled to reverse to youth, beauty, intelligence, and health. Sooner or later, the goal of social equality will be replaced by its biological and physiological counterpart: equal rights to longevity, to the sense of well-being, perhaps to resurrection (N. Fedorov).[15]

Part IV
THE NEW SCIENCE

Complementary, my dear Watson, complementary!

I

Longevity plus a sense of well-being—these are the great goals of our time. But they cannot be given adequate consideration while everyone's attention is fixed on fashionable, ambiguous problems such as "population explosion" and "pollution," woes that cannot be taken care of with traditional measures anyhow. Surprisingly, in the light of new discoveries, they find their solution, or often simply cease to exist! Our contemporary impasses are ghosts, the remnants and shadows of fossilized, semiscientific concepts that perhaps in previous eras corresponded to enlightened reasoning—but not any more.

These ghosts, these two contemporary monsters that allegedly threaten our future, preoccupy mainly the educated, well-meaning city dweller, distracting him from the true commitments of our time.

With regard to the population explosion the reasoning goes that "If we do not take drastic measures, if we permit the population increase to continue at its present rate, the world population will double or triple within the next decade and we will all suffocate or die from starvation." This is logical and therefore it is pure fantasy. Why should this growth continue without halt? By the same token we could expect a child to grow indiscriminately: If it became taller by one foot in one year, deduce that it will add ten feet in the next ten years.

As a matter of fact the population growth for the last decade did not achieve the proportions predicted by our pseudo-experts and Nobel Prize laureates. In some countries it even decreased to dangerously low levels. In the nineteen-thirties, economist L. Brentano calculated that if every human being on earth would be allotted one square meter and all of the earth's inhabitants arranged one next to the other, they would just about cover the Bodensee (a lake at the border between Germany and Switzerland). The rest of our planet would remain unoccupied.

Social groups that have achieved a certain cultural level and

93

affluence value comfort above all and automatically cut down the number of their progeny. Thus, in the last analysis, self-limitation in reproduction becomes a question of education and living standard (not of governments interfering with bedroom habits).

History tells us of nations that, after dynamically increasing in size and achieving a certain degree of maturity, culture, and wealth, began to shrink, fade, and finally completely disappeared from the scene. This trend is already at work in some contemporary Western European nations.

In many ways the entire group of nations and races can be regarded as one human tribe, one huge family that, after its infancy, adolescence, and maturity, may begin to decline and lose its miraculous capacity for propagation. So, after many annoying pregnancies, a married couple suddenly finds itself sterile and impotent; yet only a little while ago they lived in continuous fear, counting the days to the wife's next period. Such a "menopause" is the probable fate not only of separate nations but of our entire human family (unless some day it encounters a new "family" with whom it will be able to interchange seeds).

So much for the straight prediction of our highly specialized demographs. As for the argument that, meanwhile, food is becoming scarce, this too can hardly be considered valid. Deserts are still uncultivated and unirrigated; we have not even begun to exploit the sea plankton and the ocean bed. Possibilities for new energies of practically the magnitude of a *perpetuum mobile* are emerging. Nature itself is a kind of *perpetuum mobile*; the production of sugar by light (photosynthesis) is limitless, if we consider not only our sun but all the other luminous bodies in space.

Organized life in our universe is scarce. Even if there are intelligent beings somewhere, they cannot be too numerous. No, we are rather an exception in the spaces. But even simple matter, minerals and gases, atoms and protons, are scarce in our immense and continuously expanding universe.

Attempts at compounding the total amount of matter have been made since antiquity. Archimedes came to the conclusion that "a sphere of the size attributed by Aristarkus to the sphere of the fixed stars would contain a number of grains of sand, less than 10^{63}." Now we have improved our calculations. From

Lemaitre's theory it appears that the total amount of matter in the universe is about 10^{22} the sun's mass (or 10^{12} galaxies). Another expression of this calculation is that there are 10^{79} protons and as many electrons in the entire universe.

That is all. That is all our existential richness, our vital inventory, our reserve. Nothing can be added (though parts are, up to a point, interchangeable). Of that total matter, organic substances represent only a micro-fraction of 1 percent. As to intelligent creatures, we have a right (at least for the time being) to consider them a unique phenomenon, limited to our local biosphere.

All this bears out the simple observation that matter, and not only living matter, is the most precious, sacred creation in the universe. We must combine all our spiritual, intellectual, and physical capacities to protect, cultivate, and develop it. Our historic mission is to expand, to *populate* and *pollute* empty celestial bodies that are waiting for life, for a tree to be planted, a bird to nest, a child to be born there. What can be sadder and uglier than a deserted, abandoned, always cold and dark planet?

II

This brings us to the theme of pollution that is so much in vogue now among the petit bourgeois reformists and suburban admirers of nature.

Pollution is life, life is pollution; life is caused by pollution and causes it. A radical, indiscriminate fight against pollution would be a fight against life itself. (Basically it is the homosexual manifestation of our time. Aren't the antipollutionists hundred percent backers of the loop, the pill, and abortion? Apparently the lava of pornography does not pollute the brain and does not call for censorship—but a newborn child that threatens our comfort is considered pollution.)

Life, even if it is limited to our planet, is still an expression of all the cosmic forces that converge from the universe and "pollute" the earth. Correspondingly, whatever we do on our globe (which is also a celestial body) reflects on the entire cosmos and inseminates it. (V. Vernadsky).[19a]

The appearance of carbon dioxide (CO_2) was of course pollution. But without it—and water—the plants would not be able to achieve photosynthesis. Photosynthesis is accomplished with the help of light from the cosmos. This too is pollution, since too much sun is dangerous. Due to photosynthesis sugar is produced and oxygen eliminated, thrown out as a side product. This is our sole natural source of oxygen: thus even oxygen is technically speaking a product of metabolic waste, of elimination, of pollution. The fact that this particular product turned out to be beneficial to us does not change its nature. Remnants of dead organisms, of extinct animals, of vegetation, crustacea, rotting wood, polluted the earth's crust and created the conditions favorable for agriculture, animal husbandry, and deposits of coal, oil, natural gases. The marks left by digging rodents from earliest geological times; the constructions of the so-called social creatures such as beavers, ants, termites; the firm ground created by corals and seaweed; all these are manifestations of pollution that we have, so far, gratefully accepted and exploited. Mushrooms, fungi, innumerable microscopical parasites, bacteria, viruses, cause fermentation, decay, and other chemical processes that are in fact forms of pollution and yet so important that without them we may say life would cease. The priests, physicians, philosophers of antiquity, already claimed that life originates from dirt. (The cloaca is an adequate place for propagation.)

Interchanges of chemical elements brought about by volcanic eruptions played a colossal (and favorable) role in the geology of our planet. So did interchanges of solid, liquid, and gaseous masses provoked by atmospheric precipitations, by floods, sea currents, winds, and of course by migration of animals, birds, insects. The ecologists are aware of and accept all this, but do not realize that basically these processes were all forms of pollution.

There is yet another source of interchange, migration (pollution) that has come to play an enormous role in the life of our planet—and beyond it. This is the interchange ("migration") of atoms, accomplished by civilized mankind in the last century. New, unheard-of metals in pure and free state were formed by us for the first time. The new environment created by our industries infiltrates gradually the entire universe. And this may have great and beneficial effects in future eons.

No one will deny that there exist certain temporary dangers from massive pollution of our waters and backyards. It could indeed cause grave, if transitory, complications. However our cities and centers have always been polluted in one way or another since antiquity. (What were the great epidemics of the Middle Ages and Renaissance if not manifestations of pollution?)

One cannot tell a society "Don't pollute!" It is as hopeless as saying "Don't fornicate! Abstain!" Such orders work only for individuals, never for the masses. The only solution is as quickly as possible to find exhaust channels and access to new free areas. Of course we will have to pass through a critical period. But human life is never perfectly balanced; equilibrium is very rare in nature. The truth is that we must be "pushed" by some emergency toward those free areas. And those areas are immense; they lie open, they are waiting for us.

The question whether there is life outside our planet is absurd, idle, devoid of meaning. We are part of the cosmos, and what is going on here has, besides its local interest, a cosmic implication. Is there life in the cosmos? Of course there is! We are here—and we belong to the cosmos. Consciously or subconsciously we have already started to accomplish our great mission of expanding, infecting, inseminating, "polluting" the universe. This is the meaning of our history.

III

The expansion into space will not only solve scientific, demographical, ecological problems but also influence our entire mentality. A striking phenomenon could be observed during the Apollo II expedition to the moon. A report by the police authorities stated that during this period crime in the metropolitan area practically ceased. What a way of fighting crime, addiction, madness, suicidal tendencies! And yet this "indirect" approach makes sense.

The noosphere (or biosphere) is an infinitesimally thin

membrane on the crust of our earth, infected (polluted) with life and behaving as if it were meant to invade the entire universe. If in the course of this process pollution gets out of hand for a short time, it is no final catastrophe and will be gradually remedied thanks to the marvelous recuperative forces of nature. After all, we had earthquakes, floods, tidal waves, collisions of satellites and comets, migration of ice, monsters, and vegetation. It all passed by and is forgotten. Scorched islands lost in the oceans flourish again.

Suffice it to bear in mind that one diatom, a microscopic algae, if dividing unopposed, can in eight days produce a mass of matter equal to the volume of our planet, and in the next hour after that it will have doubled its mass. We ought to catapult such organisms into space, pollute our solar system with oxygen, water, carbon dioxyde, etc., etc. Foolishly we keep a strict regime for absolute sterility in all our expeditions "out." We are not particular about contaminating the Hudson or the Pacific, but it is taboo to do it to the moon or, eventually, to Mars. We are going there; whether we plan it or not, we will be there (we are there). We must settle there, not just make ten steps. The order of the day is to pollute and populate other celestial bodies.

But, instead, under the old, outlived concepts of closed systems, we have come to a completely opposite and extremely barbarian solution. As a decisive step in the fight with our contemporary evils we have finally legalized abortion. There is a logic in this absurdity. It is the logic of ignorance.

The "liberal" abortion law recently passed in New York is a frightening example of how cannibalism can evolve from pseudoscience and pseudo-progress, and it reflects the deep confusion of our times. (Its evil implications will remain with us long after the law has been revised or abolished.)

The law comprises abortions for pregnancies up to twenty-four weeks gestation (six months!). It is based on the false assumption that a fetus of six months is not alive, not "humanly" alive—whatever that means. Who gave our legislators such precise information about life? Where did they explore the nature of life? It is good to bear in mind that the greatest philosophers, naturalists, biologists, physiologists, have not arrived at a definition of life and do not know the precise borderline between the mineral kingdom and organic substances. In fact this line of demarcation is becoming more and more vague and elastic with the advance of contemporary biochemistry.

Heraclitus said that "the people should fight for the law as for their city walls." Apparently they could feel proud about their city and its legislation.

As a matter of fact it is impossible to check on a woman or on a raving adolescent who claims that she is "only" six months pregnant. There are no objective signs to distinguish between twenty-four and twenty-eight weeks of gestation. Cases were reported where such "unliving" creatures, taken out from their mothers' bellies, cried, breathed, even lived for a while. "The director of Maternity and Newborn Services for the City Department of Health said yesterday that twenty-six fetuses had remained alive after legal abortion in the cities since July. Most lived only for a few minutes, said Dr. Jean Parker, although one survived and was placed for adoption. Several of the fetuses were beyond the twenty-four week gestation period which is the legal limit for abortion here." And Dr. Parker adds that no crying fetuses who were aborted were "dropped into surgical trash cans" (*New York Times*, Dec. 19, 1970).

These operations were not performed by criminals, illiterate brutes, fascists, Hitlerists, or communists, but by middle-class intellectuals with university diplomas and a respect for the law. If it were illegal they wouldn't do it. But since the law permits it—what is the problem? Thus, many honorable Germans participated in Hitler's Vernichtungsaktionen because the experts told them that some nations are not human. They would never have done it if it were against the law. No harm came to the Japanese because the experts listed them as Aryans.

All this is the result of pseudoscience, outdated concepts, unrevised, antiquated knowledge. We have a post-nuclear technology. To handle it adequately we must acquire a post-nuclear mentality as well. Our philosophy is old-fashioned, permeated by Newton, Descartes, Darwin, Marx. Such discrepancy is potentially catastrophic.

The thesis no longer needs a fighting antithesis to become a synthesis. In the post-nuclear era, free, spontaneous jumps are quite justified and the order of the day. Consequently, we can proceed *directly* to our ideal, skipping the intermediary Hegelian stages. No more overcoming: immediate transformation or rather transfiguration is possible, we know.

IV

The sciences are based on great concepts that have emerged at different stages of our quest for knowledge. Such concepts are gravitation, cause-and-effect phenomena, thermodynamics with entropy, and, last but not least, evolution. For a long time our civilization has rested happily on these notions, but recently they have undergone drastic changes and are no longer the same.

"The scientific bases of these older discussions have been washed away and with their disappearance have gone all the arguments, such as they were, that seemed to require the acceptance of materialism and determinism and the renunciation of human free will."[20] Are we aware that these old arguments have been "washed away"?

A detailed analysis of the radical changes that occurred in our basic scientific concepts is imperative.

Since Newton, the idea of gravitation has become implanted in our reasoning. Under the impact of new experiments, data, and observations, however, the laws of Newton had to be altered or had to acquire new meaning. His formulas have become ambiguous. The law of gravitation refers to the product of the masses of the two bodies involved ($m1 \cdot m2$); but the mass depends on the velocity of the body—a fact established by Einstein. What are we to take for our formula—the changing mass of the planet under variable velocity or, perhaps, the mass reduced to rest?

The distance of the masses, also referred to in Newton's law, is connected with the observer and, thus, relative. Are we to place the observer on the sun or on the other body or at rest in the ether? Or in some other gravitational medium?

In order to explain how gravitation acts, Newton had to support the notion of an ether. If the ether, or something similar, does not exist, how does the gravitational force act on distance without an intermediary?

New concepts of a curved space-time unity were introduced that seemed to satisfy our observations. But this changed our idea of time and space (on which all psychological theories or perception were, and *still are*, based).

In addition, the notion of mass had to be modified and the theory of fields came into being. The fields simulate properties of moving masses in space: they are themselves expanded matter and carry energy (or angular momentum).

How do all these new phenomena affect our life on the cellular, molecular, nuclear level? This question has, as yet, not been answered in physiology, medicine, or sociology; we still play with the old notions.

The gravitational law, one of the basic laws from the beginning of scientific enlightenment, has influenced all fields of our culture. Some writer, for instance, suggested recently that the famous *principle of check and balance*, expressed in the American Constitution, is a direct consequence of the Newtonian gravitational concept. The change of such a concept ought then to have far-reaching repercussions. The new idea of time interferes decisively with the cause-and-effect sequence. "The present instant properly speaking does not extend beyond here. . . . The only really simultaneous events are events which occur at the same place."[21]

Cause also travels with a definite velocity that cannot exceed the speed of light (*in vacuo*). We can imagine a situation with no causal connection possible, for the speed of the connection would have to exceed the speed of light. In that case the temporal sequence of two events will be reversed (if the observer is subject to the appropriate motion). "Of two watches we have no right to say that the one goes true, the other wrong; we can only say that it is advantageous to conform to the indication of the first."[22]

We are far removed from Newton's naive definition that "absolute and mathematical time in itself and from its own nature flows equally without relation to anything external" (*Principia*). In our day, such a statement can only cause bewildered laughter. If time flowed it would itself consist of a series of events moving in time—which is utter nonsense. And what central force would control time in its uniformly equal flow, everywhere and ever? To speak of *absolute* time now is rather confusing.

But if our ideas of matter, space, and time have changed radically, little remains of Newton's image of reality.

V

The two laws of thermodynamics occupy the key position in our scientific concepts. Why these particular laws should have been expanded to such colossal dimensions is a mystery—a psychological mystery!

It is a strange paradox that the two laws to which we ascribe the greatest universality, the law of conservation of energy and the law of fatal increase of entropy, are nothing but ordinary elaborations of a simple branch of physics, thermodynamics. What an inflated career.

The modern physicist feels very uncomfortable about thermodynamics and its too-far-reaching generalizations. It is certainly bad manners, today, to speak of thermodynamics in the terms of the 19th century. The approach through statistical mechanics and kynetic theory is bound to give us a much deeper and less abstract insight. But, according to our school books and basic training, the two laws of thermodynamics are still absolute truth.

The first law, as it stands, is the law of conservation of energy. Its conventional differential formula is $dE = dW + dQ$. The equation is applicable to a "region" that is defined by a surface that isolates it *completely* from the surroundings. Thus this operation on the cosmic scale would demand the separation of the universe into at least two parts: one inside, whose changes of E we are tracing, and the other one outside. In addition, an *external* observer is necessary who makes the instrumental operations on the *inside* part to evaluate the change of energy (dE). From such a point of view it is meaningless to talk about the energy of the entire universe—and whether it increases or decreases—for the universe, by definition, cannot have a place outside of itself and an external observer who in no way interferes with the system inside.

All our operations in search of absolute energy give meaning only to *changes* of energy, not to energy of the initial or the final state. Thus we have only change-of-energy; and whether this corresponds to energy itself is the big question. Even if proven that the law of energy itself applies ideally to the change-of-energy, we do not know its relation to energy in general. And yet the first law of thermodynamics is the law of conservation of energy in general in the universe. And we still speak of it as a scientific concept!

We do not know the original or the final state of energy, its dimensions and its change in the universe. To postulate a law of the conservation of energy in the universe is a pseudoscientific enterprise; science based on such assumptions is not science. The discrepancy has been obvious to many good men. Yet for a certain time the law served its purpose. With the progress of physics, and since the advent of new quantum mechanics, the inherent contradictions of the law have become untenable.

Later we shall see that the heat produced by work can never be wholly reversed into work again. If this holds true it means that, for all practical purposes, an amount of energy is lost. On the other hand, constant *new* sources of new energies seem to arise spontaneously through new universal cataclysms, according to modern observations. Such a fact is in flagrant contradiction to the old dictum of thermodynamics. Yet, in our mentality, in everyday life, in the fields of conventional art, law, medicine and the social sciences, this dictum still persists as a basic concept and exerts its influence on our conscience.

VI

We know already that the notion of reversibility, as well as irreversibility, is one of the cardinal points in science. Little however can be found in the textbooks concerning their meaning. Medical references only list irreversibility. Gould, for instance, says: (1) not capable of being reversed; (2) irrevocable; (3) said of a state of shock or nerve injury from which recovery cannot be achieved.

This is all. Not much, considering that an attempt at deliberating along these lines could shed some light upon the basic problems of medicine. After all, a great part if not all of the medical art could be defined as an attempt to reverse some natural or pathological process.

The "exact" sciences pay more attention to the complex nature of irreversibility. Physicists of all schools speculate on the subject. The best way to explore the problem is perhaps to use Planck's illustration.[23]

A piece of heated iron is immersed in cold water. It passes on its heat to the water until both reach the same temperature, the so-called thermal equilibrium that always results unless conduction of heat is prevented. The flow is always *in one direction*, from hot to cold, and therefore represents an irreversible process.

In another operation, two glass tubes, open at the upper ends, are connected at their lower openings by a rubber tube; if some heavy liquid—for instance, mercury—is poured into one tube, it flows through the rubber into the second tube, rising until the level in both tubes is equal. When one of the tubes is lifted the level becomes disturbed, but when the tube is lowered to the initial position, the fluid returns to the previous level. This is reversibility par excellence.

VII

The concept of entropy arose from the irreversible processes of thermodynamics. Entropy is the measure of the disorganization of the system. Where entropy increases order diminishes; chance is creeping in, so that conditions become chaotic. The disorganization of a system may even become complete (although this is very slow in manifesting itself) and the state reached will be the irreversible thermodynamic equilibrium. Entropy cannot grow farther, since the second law of thermodynamics allows a decrease in temperature only if there is a *difference* in temperature between two bodies or mediums. Thus entropy, at that absolute point, remains forever constant; it cannot increase any further. One of the universal signposts for the direction of time thus disappears: here, in this particular system, time ceases! For time is measured by the constant increase of entropy. A state of thermodynamic equilibrium (if such does exist) is necessarily a state of absolute death. The fight against all forms of death is, basically, a fight against the second law of thermodynamics.

Entropy, we said, is determined by the amount of "disorder" in a system. However, it is a very strange notion of disorder. Let's assume we shuffle a pack of cards and then claim that the cards had—or had not—been "well shuffled." Can we describe the shuffling as good before the cards have been dealt? Or should we see the hand before saying that it was well shuffled? It is natural to say that in good shuffling the cards are put into disorder, that is, with no apparent sequence. But whether the cards are in this sort of disorder can be told only by an inspection of the hand, not merely by observing the process of shuffling. Also, it is clear that the rules of a game may always be formulated in such a way as to make any given arrangement into a favorable "sequence" for the given game. "Disorder" has nothing absolute about it; it depends on the convention of the game. And yet, the classical concept is that the more we shuffle the cards the more "disorder" occurs: entropy increases—and is irreversible; it is impossible to reestablish the previous order of the cards by continuing to shuffle them ad infinitum (or it is highly improbable).

The most outstanding feature of our universe is the continuous creation of material structures of an extremely high degree of orderliness. A man, a fly, a bacterium, a fungus, are highly ordered and *therefore* most improbable structures; that is, highly unlikely to have been created by shaking *at random* the requisite number of different kinds of atoms in a test tube. According to some thinkers, the appearance and evolution of organic life is a flagrant negation of the second law of thermodynamics that makes an increase in entropy (or disorder) mandatory and continuous. The classic riposte that, in order to continue living and growing and multiplying indefinitely, these structures have to metabolize and to take up energy from their surroundings to a degree that raises the *total* entropy beyond the *locally* achieved organization—this classic answer does not seem to exhaust the subject. By what outsider, and by what means was this amount of energies (inside an isolated system!) calculated and the correct comparison made? Is it not possible to claim that a human being capable of creating what it did create, and of appreciating it as well, may be far superior in orderliness as compared to the energy used up by it in forms of minerals, gases, and radiations? It is worth mentioning here that some modern theories claim that our universe is not a closed (isolated) one, that there are spontaneous interrelations with other "cosmic oceans" of energy (Dirak).[45]

Obviously science is now at that crucial point where a wide range of new observations and important experiences claim a completely new theoretical interpretation. Consciously or subconsciously, humanity has, throughout history, challenged irreversibility and disorder. It appears that there are enough data available to override the second law of thermodynamics with its far-reaching generalizations.

VIII

Most of the fanatic exponents of entropy and heat death adhere to the opinion that the universe "has always existed." To allow for the world to have been created in time would admit the concept of an unprecedented, spontaneous, undetermined act, perhaps even a deus ex machina. They simply ignore the fact that, if the universe exists from infinity, with entropy increasing steadily, inexorably, irreversibly, the final stage of heat death should have already been attained.

The probability that a stone will fall upwards or that temperature will flow from lower to upper level is so fantastically small that we disregard it completely. The same for reversibility of any of the so-called irreversible processes. And yet, if we knew that such a case had occurred even *once* in the history of the universe, it would change our outlook completely. If we were to forget the science of aeronautics, it would take us thousands of years to again construct a machine that, being heavier than air, could fly. But if all along we were aware that it had already been done once, that ages ago some brothers Wright did for a moment or an hour fly, the entire problem would appear in a different light. (Herein lies the importance of the case of Lazarus.)

As Sir Oliver Lodge stated in a discussion before the British Association of Scientists in 1931: "The final and inevitable increase of entropy to a maximum is a bug-bear, an idol, to which philosophers need not bow the knee."

In 1827, Robert Brown described the movement of particles that since bears his name. This movement, this famous "dance," grew wilder if the temperature of the medium rose; with temperature falling, the movement slowed and, the force of gravitation exerting its own influence, most of the particles slowly floated toward the bottom.

According to classical thermodynamics, the most probable place for the particles ought to be the bottom of the recipient. However, once at the bottom, the particles do not rest peacefully; hit by the liquid's molecules, they begin to move and, as there is no more way down, rise a little, fall, rise, in a kind of *perpetuum mobile*. In short, a reversibility in the processes of thermodynamics manifests itself. "The absolute partisan of thermodynamics would consider it a miracle if stones, thrown down to the bottom, would by themselves begin to move and rise back from the ground. But here, under the microscope, we see how this miracle constantly occurs."[24]

The explanation may lie in the concept of fluctuation. Despite a thermodynamic equilibrium in the universe, fluctuation still occurs in different parts of the system (our part of the universe may be the result of such a fluctuation). It is precisely this unequal distribution of energy that is the condition for the genesis of life and mankind. This fluctuation may vanish, but inevitably other fluctuations will appear in different parts of the cosmos. Thus some universes perish, others come into being. In such a cosmos there is no absolute direction of time, because all processes are reversible. ("The direction of time and entropy exists only inside the fluctuations"—L. Boltzman, *Laws of Gases.*)

We see that thermic death, final entropy, and irreversibility belong to only one, perhaps completely outdated, school of thought. There are, in mathematics and physics, philosophies based on new concepts. Yet biology, medicine, sociology, continue to be based on the old thermodynamics that necessarily leads to a fictitious irreversible dead end with all its agonizing implications.

According to the third law of thermodynamics, entropy goes to zero at zero (absolute) degrees; therefore, there can be no disorder left at that temperature. Thus, at absolute zero temperature, a *perpetuum mobile* can come into being. What a paradox! At zero absolute temperature a self-maintained heat engine can be indefinitely run, in flagrant violation of thermodynamics. Suppose, some day, a human being will build such a machine—an infinite source of newly created energy.

"Thus if one computes the zero point energy due to quantum mechanical fluctuation in even one cubic centimeter of space, one comes out with something of the order of 10^{38} ergs which is equal to that which would be liberated by fission of about 10^{10} tons of uranium."[25]

The new cosmology admits the possibility that the nature of the universe requires continuous creation, a perpetual bringing into being of new background materials! The fact that we do not know from where the created material comes or that it seems to come from nowhere is no argument against it. Material may simply emerge, denying our common sense: It is created.

It appears that the development of the universe in time leads to an inexhaustible diversity of new sources of energy. It is not energy that is lacking nor gold nor food nor space for the Indians and Puerto Ricans. Our crisis stems from the failure to acknowledge and make use of those infinite oceans of energy.

It is appropriate here to note that those idealistic and pseudoscientific groups that are now fighting against the pollution of seas and rivers are almost all partisans of population control, not realizing that those contraceptives that interfere with the intimate rhythm of woman's nature pollute the very sources of our life.

A reevaluation of the human status in a universe so rich in energy and so scarce in organic life is of prime necessity. Our crisis is a philosophical (or a spiritual), not an economic one.

IX

Law and joy were reigning in the kingdom of science, since Newton introduced his mathematics into physics of the sky. Common sense was joined to science, and now superior intelligence could explain anything anywhere. Mankind listened to the high priests of science and applauded. Cause and effect dictated the course of nature and its history. Laplace proclaimed: "We may regard the present state of the universe as the effect of its past and the cause for its future. An intelligence which at a given moment knew all the forces that animate nature and the respective positions of the beings that compose it, and further possessing the scope to analyze this data, could condense into a single formula the movement of the greatest bodies of the universe and that of the last atom; for such an intelligence nothing could be uncertain, and past and future alike would be before its eyes." Words such as these were supposed to represent rational science as opposed to religious mysticism.

Unfortunately, this clear-cut idea of a complete and unbroken determinism had to be demolished by the discovery of quanta and by the deep implications of this discovery. Modern scientists have come to recognize, very slowly and much against their own will, the impossibility of furnishing coherent causal descriptions of the happenings on the atomic scale.

"In the general problem of quantum theory one is faced not with a modification of the theories describable in terms of usual physical concepts, but with an essential failure of the pictures in space and time on which the description of natural phenomena has hitherto been based."[27]

Then came Heisenberg's uncertainty relation. When we want to "see" a particle—electron, proton, nucleon—we must illuminate it with the help of radiation of extremely short wavelength. The shorter the wavelength the more energetic the radiation. To be able to observe a particle we must, therefore, bombard it with high-energy photons that, after having hit the target, rebound with diminished energy and are reflected into the eye of the observer or onto a photographic plate. This is when the catastrophe occurs: the disturbance suffered by the particle in its collision with the photon changes the particle's position: to see an electron is to interfere with its movement. The radiation of extremely short wavelength hits the particle and alters its velocity, forcing it into a zig-zag course (side effect). Even worse—actually, we cannot speak of the same particle any more. Two observations, even if following each other in rapid succession, are in fact disconnected events and cannot justifiably be combined into a single comprehensive picture. Nor is there any way of telling what happened between the two observations. In short, any picture of reality on the atomic level must, by implication, contain gaps that cannot be filled in. Any attempt at tracing the path of an atomic particle *must* fail. Either we are not certain about its position (p) or we have changed its velocity (q). This is Heisenberg's *uncertainty relation*, one of the dominant principles of atomic physics: $dp \cdot dq = h$ (h = Planck's universal constant).

The question of whether the particle, twice observed, is really and truly the same is not only undecidable but also completely devoid of meaning. To put the question like that is naive. As Heisenberg said: "Atoms possess geometrical qualities in no higher degree than color or taste." Just as we reproached the ancient religions with being animistic and investing the gods with human traits, so we must reproach science for doing exactly the same with the microcosmos by ascribing to it our macroscopic characteristics.

Physicists have always felt uneasy about the heterogenous theoretical structure that emerged from the simple juxtaposition of a continuous physics of radiation (waves) and a discontinuous physics of matter (particles). Here arose the greatest crisis: the quantum crisis.

Light consists of individual entities. The existence of light corpuscles—photons—was proven by the photoelectric effect. If a light source emitted a spherical *wave* into its surroundings, the emitted energy should be scattered through space and the influence of the light become *weaker* according to the distance. This does not correspond to reality. Here, a *corpuscular* theory of photons gives the adequate explanation: the corpuscle conserves its energy like a shell full of explosives and, whatever the distance from its source, will always produce the same effect, the *photo-electric effect*. The influence of light on atoms is the same, regardless of distance travelled through space. Here is the proof that the luminous energy is concentrated in corpuscular form.

On the other hand, correct interpretation of interference and defraction still requires the wave theory. This contradiction resulted in a dichotomy in the theory of light. The only way out of the crisis was in a simultaneous introduction of both theories of light, the continuous and the discontinuous (wave *and* particle), which changed our notion of reality completely, making it perhaps unintelligible—but nonetheless real.

This crisis reflected on the theory of matter in general, since particles on a smaller scale, like electrons within the atom, did not obey the laws classical mechanics ascribed to matter. Here also discontinuity appeared, and not only discontinuity of structure but also discontinuity of motion. Within atoms, an internal state of stability would remain for lengthy periods and then, suddenly, spontaneously, a transfer by jump into another state would occur (like mutation on the evolutionary scale). It seemed impossible to explain such a transition in terms of classical theories. The question arose whether our ideas of time and space as a perfectly continuous framework of reality were genuinely valid at the atomic level.

That was the crisis that shook the entire structure of modern knowledge. It had its repercussions in every field confronting the continuous and the discontinuous aspects of reality (but medical and social sciences have not responded to it, as yet).

Thus the theory known as wave mechanics came into being, pioneered by de Broglie. "The fundamental idea is that it is essential to introduce *simultaneously* the notion of the corpuscle and that of the wave."[28]

X

The quantum state is a completely new state, different from that of objects of large dimensions. It behaves dualistically: it is a wave and a particle, not a wave and not a particle, and still something else. This is new. And this is important to us since biology, too, proceeds on a microscopic level.

Niels Bohr, who did most for the clarification of this new reality, introduced a special term, his famous *complementarity*. The two descriptions of the atom—the wavelike quantum state and the planetary model of a particle—are complementary descriptions, each true as long as applied separately. We can describe atomic reality only by telling truthfully what happens when we observe a phenomenon in *different* ways, although it may seem incredible to us that the same electron can behave as differently as it appears to in its two complementary situations. This however does not make electrons any less concrete than any other reality we observe in nature. The quantum states of the electron are the basis of what, today, we call reality.

"Consequently evidence obtained under different experimental conditions cannot be comprehended within a single picture but must be regarded as *complementary* in the sense that only the totality of the phenomena exhausts the possible information about the objects."[29]

Thus the laws of the quantum theory require us to renounce the notion of unique and precisely defined conceptual models in favor of *complementary pairs* of loosely defined models.

For his (Bohr's) assumption, that the basic properties of matter can never be understood rationally in terms of unique and unambiguous models, implies that the use of complementary pairs of imprecisely defined concepts will be necessary for the detailed treatment of every domain that will ever be investigated. "Thus the limitations on our concepts implicit in the principle of complementarity are regarded as absolute and final."[30]

In the 17th century, Silesius put it this way: "He who would rightly comprehend the world must be now Democritus and now Heraclitus."

From the context of this chapter it seems that, henceforth,

the modern scientist need not be repulsed, a priori, by theological discussions proceeding on the level of the Nicene Creed. But scientific officialdom still feels shy. And the peculiar thing is that the less scientific—the less exact—the discipline, the more belligerent it is toward uncommon sense and "metaphysics." The nuclear physicist comes very close to theological reasoning, the biologist is more reluctant, and doctors and "social scientists" remain the most adamant and still the greatest exponents of so-called objective studies based on "empirical" data. The fact is that there is no such thing as objective science in our day.

To quote Heisenberg: "By playing with both pictures (particle and wave), by going from one picture to the other and back again, we finally get the right impression of the strange kind of reality behind our atomic experiments." It certainly is a most remarkable fact that this reality is such as to need two different and seemingly exclusive sets of concepts to describe it. There is nothing absurd in our notion of a wave-particle duality of matter. It only appears absurd if one tries to combine both aspects into a single picture. Is matter particles or waves? Answer yes or no! This is the wrong approach—the approach of our judicial procedures. Matter is particles and waves, and perhaps something else. But those aspects never manifest themselves *together* in one and the same experimental setting. Common logic will not help us. It is the uncommon that is the order of the day.

In the last analysis, reversibility and irreversibility becomes a question of probability and logic. In principle, the laws of nuclear physics have demonstrated themselves to be reversible. Any given motion and duration can, in principle, be executed in the reverse order. But such a reversal does not usually occur spontaneously, at least not within our practically observable time: it is very *improbable* that it will occur.

Into the problem of the shuffled cards or the mixed gases, the notion of probability enters. A common-sense calculation for fluctuation of two gases would show that a chance combination of motion that would lead *all* the oxygen and hydrogen back into their original containers would not occur for $10^{10^{10}}$ years (one followed by 10,000 million zeros). That is considered the end of the argument. However, the calculation of the chances for the appearance of a Mozart, in the 18th century, in central Europe,

from a molecule of hydrogen squeezed for billions of years between two nebulas beyond the Milky Way—those chances are
probably of the same order. What already has happened we are
inclined to consider natural. It would be good to assimilate—
once and for all—that the almost impossible is also almost possible (especially if the dice should be loaded—if atoms and cells
have a certain *direction* or preference).

Heat can go from a lower to a higher temperature, water can
flow back from the sea to the mountains, and time can theoreti-
cally reverse its direction.

Reality itself may not be that complex and contradictory. It
only appears to us obscure and ambiguous due to the limitations
of our perception and intelligence. Whether these limitations
must remain with us forever or whether we can still develop and
acquire new faculties is a question different schools of thought
answer in different ways. The now-fashionable philosophy of
Teilhard de Chardin (as well as some theosophical schools)
affirms the latter. Unfortunately, Teilhard also sees God as
still evolving (and, as it seems, from matter).[31]

XI

The impossibility of measuring certain quantities relating to
atomic particles is the basis of Heisenberg's uncertainty principle. Indeed, we cannot determine with full accuracy both velocity and position of an electron. This impossibility is more than a
temporary technical limitation that may, someday, be overcome.
If it were possible, someday, to perform such accurate mea-
surements, the concept of the double nature of matter—wave and
particle—would collapse, since such measurement would prove
one of the two alternatives to be wrong. Heisenberg's principle
expresses our image of the dual nature of atomic objects
forever—at least as perceived by us. If this double nature could
be denied, "our interpretation of the wide field of atomic
phenomena would become only a chain of errors with its success

based only on accidental coincidence."[32] (In other words, *the odds are against it!* Improbable—but not impossible.)

It is important to acknowledge that the phenomena studied in contemporary physics present features having no equivalent in the classical theories. We are in the process of molding a system of new concepts, which means creation of a new mode of thinking plus a new language. Art, psychology, medicine, and law must also take part in this process.

What follows from Heisenberg's principle (dp · dq = h) is that the description of atomic particles always contains an uncertainty, which is in part objective, due to the *uncertainty relation*, and in part subjective, due to our incomplete knowledge. As Heisenberg puts it: "They [the atoms] form a world of potentialities or possibilities rather than of things and facts."

The other consequence related to the above is the impossibility of predicting the result of an observation with certainty. It is only the probability that can be predicted, which means that causality ceases to operate on this level. This pulls the ground from under the Laplacian program, knocks down the basis on which it rests, namely that the state of the particles in the universe can ever be known with sufficient accuracy. It has become clear to us that the present is unknowable, cannot and never will be knowable, and that, consequently, no conclusive information with regard to the future can be drawn from available data. It is indeed a breakdown of causality that, *nolens volens*, brings us back to the old notion of free will—at least on the atomic level. It makes no sense, now, to use an expression such as "the precise path of a photon. . . ." A photon may indeed describe a precise path, but we cannot observe this. And what is more, the photon may choose one path or another: nothing can predict its free course. We do know that 70 percent of the photons will be absorbed and reflected, and this statistical knowledge does save the day for many practical purposes.

We cannot follow the behavior of one single particle on its journey in space and time, but we can try another solution. Let us assume we shoot an electron from a sort of gun, aiming always at the same spot, a photographic plate, where the impacts are meticulously recorded. We repeat this a large number of times and, on inspection, find that the points of impact lie scattered about. Exactly the same experiment is repeated over and over, and yet the result, each time, is different, fluctuating. But although each electron hits the target in a different place, the spots are arranged in an orderly way, forming a perfectly regular pattern. Thus, out of randomness, order is born. Where many electrons hit the plate, light rings appear; dark ones where none hit or only a few.

What cannot be predicted of one individual electron can be predicted of a large number, and with great accuracy. If we cease to care for the fate of a single particle and turn to that of a crowd, we regain the apparently lost faculty to predict the future and formulate its laws. Suppose a million electrons were sent in the same direction; quantum mechanics allows us to predict how many of them will hit the center, which fraction will fall on the first rings, which on the second, and so on, predictions the more accurately confirmed the larger the crowd involved.

What emerges is a *statistical* theory, unconcerned with individuals, that takes into account only large assemblages. The structure of this theory is such that statements derived from it describe the *probability* with which a particle may be found at a certain place: where in fact it will be, thereof the laws keep silent.

When sun rays hit a window, a part of the photons of which the rays consist is absorbed (or let through) while another part is reflected. If a single photon is isolated—and this can be done!—it will either go through or be reflected. There is no predicting its course. Something resembling free will is left to such units.

Physicians can only guess as to the concrete implications of this new principle of the quantum mechanics for biophysics or pathology. However, already it seems outdated when a pathologist or a geneticist stains living and isolated tissue with lethal solutions, puts it under an electron microscope, and believes that he is studying the "nature" of the cells without interference. The frozen section, on which so much in contemporary medicine is based, is an anachronism of 18th century reasoning. Even if obvious changes occurred *immediately* in a cell when cancer originates, they would be masked and distorted by our brutal interference. Insofar as we are proceeding on the nuclear level, this distortion will remain a fact, and all our knowledge of cancer will remain inadequate. Great pathologists know that structures may be already cancerous while not disclosing it through our conventional methods. Other structures show, in vitro, signs similar to cancer, yet are not always malignant. The question how this distorts our statistics has never been posed officially.

Meanwhile we still adhere in medical research to the old concept of cause and effect: he (or she) got cancer *because* he (or she) smoked; he (or she) got cured *because* all lymph glands were dissected and excised. If the nature of cancer were being studied where it ought to be, namely on the molecular and atomic levels, the indeterministic philosophy of nuclear physics would enter into the picture and perhaps break through the dead end of our outdated causal theories. (This applies to both etiology and therapy.)

A statistical theory has emerged through nuclear physics that is unconcerned with the individual case and takes into account only enormous assemblages. In medicine this principle would project itself along such lines: regardless of operative procedure, n percent of cancer patients will die within three years after operation (perhaps by their own choice, that is, choice on the cellular level).

Another example to illustrate the above: 1 mg of radium comprises a vast number of atoms of which half, we know, will have disintegrated within 10,000 years. But if we could pick out one single atom we would not be able to tell whether this particular one will be among the "10,000-year survivors" or will erupt within the next few seconds. There is no way of foretelling it, and not because of human limitations. It is objectively *uncertain* when this particular atom will come to disintegrate. We set down only statistical decrees! Thus the percentage of sexagenarians who will die next year in Florida can be predicted statistically. But not individual cases. The same applies to the five years survival after mastectomy. There is no way of telling who will survive—and whether it was a radical or simple mastectomy does not influence the outcome.

An atom of radium erupts whenever it chooses to. This is

quite literally an un-causal event. Such un-causal events must also be taking place in the field of medicine where we are now engaged in elaborations on the cellular, genetic, and atomic levels. The freedom of "eruption" and/or the freedom of choice must have its reflection on the social plane too: the boy who has murdered a gorgeous blonde did not necessarily do it *because*, many years before, he saw his mother in bed with their neighbor.

Part V
THE NEW REALITY

The dice are loaded. . . .

I

According to the second law of thermodynamics, matter disintegrates; order in the cosmos diminishes; entropy increases; zero equilibrium and death are the natural fate of the universe. Regularly, scientists convene to debate, with greater or lesser precision, this heat death, while next door evolutionists and Darwinists deliberate on the number of billions of years it took a simple cell to become man. Evolution, which is organization and order, was made possible by a process antagonistic to the second law of thermodynamics, by the build-up process, which occurred due to the phenomenon of self-replication, that is, multiplication, organization, and improvement of structures.

Scientists are aware of this contradiction and have their answer. They claim that the second law of thermodynamics with its inevitable destruction and death is still right for a closed system; within the framework of this closed system, however, a particular small sector may increase its order, build up its structure, decrease its entropy, while feeding on the entire system to which it belongs and, thus, increasing the entropy of the latter. The total measure of disorder therefore keeps increasing.

According to the conventional scientist, the increase of order in a living structure is always accompanied by a decrease of order in the sustaining physical environment: for every protein molecule constructed so much light energy is absorbed that it results in a large loss of order in the sun. And so, gradually, a sponge, a fish, a mammal, came into being; then the monkey, and the caveman, followed by Homer, Saint Francis of Assisi, and Einstein. The increase of order and organization in those latter specimens corresponds to the loss of solar energy and sustains the total increase in entropy. And yet we can imagine a planet with the same laws of thermodynamics on which plants, insects, rodents, and something very similar to man evolved, but never a Saint Paul, a Plato, or a Pascal.

Why did Christ or Buddha come into being? It is very

121

simple: "A more complicated structure appears if and when this structure is better adapted to its environment." Christ was better adapted . . . "To turn the other cheek" is the law of the fittest! Socrates who refuses to run from a cruel sentence "because we are supposed to respect the law, even a stupid and unjust law." These are the fittest, for they survived and will be alive and influencing us as long as one man on our earth is still able to read and think.

On the other hand, any bully or ape or successful executive who devours his neighbor and takes over his office (or hut) is also the fittest, for apparently he survives. By simultaneously playing two hands (even *and* odd, red *and* black), the old scientist cannot lose. Perhaps he cannot win either, this way.

The Marxist explains the humanitarian line in our culture by means of the psychological overstructure: A class that has become rich and assured of its future *always* evolves a mentality with some idealistic tendencies. This is why the Russian revolution was primarily prepared by noblemen and bourgeois (not by the muzhiks and the workers). Here again, by interpreting miraculous results in their deterministic way, 18th-century-inspired philosophers can always appear to be the winners.

If our organic and cultural life is only a lately added small appendix to the dying-out universe, it is possible to accept such a point of view. But if the organic world and our Western civilization, marked miraculously by a concept of love and light, is not a small added afterthought, not a simple episode but an immense, infinite phenomenon, then the entire elaboration of the second law of thermodynamics appears as a contradition: A greater part cannot feed on a smaller!

To us this is of tremendous significance, since "to turn the other cheek" represents a process of complete reversibility of the course of natural events and a negation of our cause-and-effect dictum. This brings us to Darwinism or to what our contemporary scientists are forced to call neo-Darwinism in an attempt to gloss over the all-too-obvious contradictions.

II

No natural scientist now accepts the classical theory of evolution as it was presented in the 19th century. Numerous changes and adjustments are constantly being made. The notion of the fittest was revised, genetics added, Lamarck in massive doses rehabilitated. In fact, a new theory of evolution has emerged during the last decades that, for sentimental reasons, is called neo-Darwinism (by the same token it could have been called neo-Lamarckism or even neo-Mendelism).

Darwin did not suspect the existence of an entire field of modern science, namely genetics with its mutations and *sudden* jumps. He could have read Mendel's article, which appeared in 1866 in a second-rate Austrian magazine and was ignored by all the great men of the time. Rediscovered at the beginning of the 20th century, it became the cornerstone of a new concept in evolution. To that the neo-Darwinists added greater portions of Lamarck's theory of environmental influence (while the concept of sexual adaptation became almost obliterated).

The main point of Darwinism lies in its chance element, which from the start brought many skeptical reactions. Darwin tried to prove that species reproduce themselves with some *minute* deviations: for nature cannot exactly copy itself, just as a gun cannot always hit precisely the same spot on the target. "*Natura non facit saltum.*" This is wrong. It might explain the occurrence of new variations but never of new species. (Mutations are jumps—spontaneous, unprecedented, and perhaps undetermined.)

Some of those minute Darwinian changes are viable, others not. The nonviable are automatically wiped out by Mother Nature and good neighbors. The viable forms adapt themselves to the environment, meet some other successful survivors, and produce new variations that in turn, if viable, continue to establish themselves, slowly but surely, first as varieties and then as new *species*. Thus, according to Darwin, are old species transformed and new ones generated.

As a general result, the organic world evolves from the simplest rudimentary forms to the most complicated and perfect, with man the crowning glory. Odd, that this automatic, blind killing of everything around that can be killed should result in an *assured* general—physical, intellectual, spiritual—improvement. Odd, that this blind natural law should be directed only one way, toward complication, organization, perfection, and humanization. Is it really blind and aimless, acting—as it does—as if it had an inner tendency toward some goal, namely self-reproduction (and perhaps in a better, more perfect form)? This is the least we can say now, without any danger of being excommunicated by the high priests of science. In all safety we may state: "The cells act as if they had a *tendency* to reproduce themselves." By introducing "as" and "if," the scientists hope to avoid the immense controversy that would arise from attributing a tendency to a cell: This would be metaphysics! And yet, if we could admit the existence of a general force or a tendency—universal, like gravitation—in the cell, everything around us would become clear and comprehensible. But the old scientist cannot admit such a tendency, even though all reality points toward it; he cannot accept it, lest he permit metaphysics to slip into so-called objective science. He cannot permit it, conditioned as he is by the 18th century philosophy of science that does not recognize metaphysics and accepts only one dictum: cause and effect—this fetish of common sense.

Here is the crisis: allegiance to a fossilized, 18th-century philosophy that stands in the way of new, great discoveries. The fact is that Darwin himself and many of his followers had certain doubts about the very foundations of Darwinism, such as natural selection, sexual selection, and the so-called survival of the fittest. For reasons that cannot be analyzed here, but that undoubtedly have a firm psychological basis, the average naturalist, biologist, and above all the intellectuals of all species and fields did not pay any attention to the doubts and remorse of Darwin. Here is a confession by the latter: ". . . but I now admit . . . that in the earlier editions of my *Origin of Species* I probably attributed too much to the action of natural selection or the survival of the fittest . . . I had not formerly sufficiently considered the existence of many structures which appear to be, as far as we can judge, neither beneficial nor injurious; and this I believe to be one of the greatest oversights as yet detected in my work."[33]

No one paid due attention to his confession. The Darwinists were eager to join the bandwagon—with or without their chief. And since then, this dance macabre of the survival of the fittest, as the basis for progress, has been part of our scientific and intellectual luggage.

In an attempt to correct the contradictions of the theory of the "fittest," and reluctant to give due credit to environmental influences in evolution (which were Lamarck's findings), Darwin introduced and fully exploited the notion of sexual selection. However, it is a fact that the display of their sexual characteristics rather handicaps the species in their everyday struggle for life and exposes them to the enemy. The famous peacock fan, so tempting, apparently, in courtship, is probably a nuisance in competing for food or in warding off a foe. Elaborate courting procedures make some species more vulnerable and even prone to genetic disturbances.

In *The Descent of Man*, Darwin writes: "Mr. V. Kovalevsky informs me from Russia that he noticed bloodcovered patches on the snow where the woodcocks had fought; when several woodcocks engage in fierce battle their feathers fly in all directions." And further: "Mr. Kovalevski insists that the females sometimes steal away with a young cock who dare not enter the fight against the older males just so as it does happen with the great stags in Scotland."[34] Our contemporaries leave no doubt about their opinion on the subject: As Konrad Lorenz puts it "For the rest, I believe that our experience with *captive* animals and, of course, with our own species, misleads us into overestimating the loss of individuals incurred by intraspecific fighting in most animals."

And yet, what romantic repercussions these theories of "fights" and "fittest" had on our mentality, on life, the arts, and even politics. A young gentleman in the Indian jungle, building the British Empire with an iron fist, could be certain that, in the last analysis, all his cruelty served progress, evolution, and humanity. The influence of scientific and pseudoscientific theories (Darwin's, Marx's, Freud's, Pavlov's) has been catastrophic. Especially since they attracted primarily people ignorant in these fields.

Some butterflies take on the gray appearance of tree leaves "in order to survive"; others manifest the most striking colors as if to advertise: we are poisonous, do not touch us; others again remain in between, not really garish, yet not gray either—and all survive. The moths fly irrationally into fire or light and also survive, in spite of it.

When a species has died off or when it has established itself in time, it is always easy, post factum, to find a reason for it. And this reason may be the same for both cases, though it did lead to opposite results. The ancestors of the giraffe who increased the length of their necks by a fraction of a centimeter at a time, through the centuries, could not possibly have profited from it in their fight for survival; they must have "known" through some revelation that eventually their long neck would be an asset. A possum plays dead, a cat grows sharp teeth and claws, an elk develops a fast pace—all "defend" themselves in different ways. Are these not reflections of their personal choices, sympathies, and preferences? A skunk became a skunk, perhaps, because he liked and wanted to be one.

Wasps, bees, and hornets sting in order to defend themselves, and, afterwards, some die. A strange way of self-defense! But thus they save perhaps their community? Yes. Though the defense of one's community by an act of personal sacrifice is quite different from the free-for-all of "survival." Why did an infusorium continue to evolve, when it was practically immortal?

III

The numerous inner weaknesses of Darwin's theory appear in all aspects and layers of his work. The principle of the survival of the fittest is, to say the least, an ambiguous notion. Is it not rather so that the one who survived is recognized as the fittest *because* he has survived (similar to the notion of disorder in thermodynamics as applied to a beautifully organized crystal)? Many Darwinists recognize the shortcomings of this mainstay of the theory. Some now claim that it is enough just to be "fit," to survive (T. Dobzhansky, *Mankind Evolving*). But the fit is not the fittest—so that the very foundation of the theory of evolution through natural selection (of the superior, the fittest) is destroyed; for there is no opportunity left for natural selection to operate and produce a *fitter* form, variety, or species.

Also, the struggle for existence has a retarding effect as well on the species. Selye's theory of stress applies much more to animals than to man. The fittest, after some time of struggle and stress, becomes less fit (deteriorates) and offers ever fewer prospects for procreation and the emergence of new, *fitter* forms.

Like the survival of the fittest, the famous struggle for existence is also a half truth that, blown up into an exclusive truth, becomes a lie. Of course there is a struggle for existence! However, the new species comes into being not due to this struggle but in spite of it: The greater the struggle for existence, the more slowly evolution proceeds.[35]

Many authors, before and after Darwin, have written about cooperation among insects and animals. Here again we come up against that psychological block that makes the average scientist, biologist, intellectual, ignore those studies having no sensational appeal for the imagination. The less we are able to live an active life, the more attracted we are to the epical "kill or be killed." The same psychological law that directs the "common people" away from Proust or Kafka toward books and plays where one fellow with two pistols advances against the enemy's camp— this same law pushes the great intellectuals toward the mythical struggle for survival, far removed from the reality of cooperation and tolerance in life. Yet it is a fact that mutual aid and support eliminate a great deal of competition in nature.[36]

What everybody wants from life is the greatest possible fullness and intensity, with the least amount of time and energy wasted on mere essentials. Woods and prairies, where killers of all species choke each other incessantly and tenaciously, are a romantic dream. The jungles are "so favorable that almost anything can survive and almost anything does."[37] As for the arctic, Stephenson has written at length about the friendliness of that region.

Love and solidarity are perhaps at the basis of our evolution, not competition and struggle. "I think there has been an increasing tendency in biological writing to stress the cooperative rather than the competitive aspect of relations among various kind of organisms. But this tendency has not been adequately reflected in the thinking of the social philosophers who have tended to confine their biological explorations to the post-Darwinian or Thomas Huxley period. I don't think the social philosophers are entirely to be blamed for this. The biologists have failed to make their growing knowledge, their accumulating facts and concepts easily available to the philosophers."[38]

Although no naturalist will speak of evolution in terms of Darwin and Huxley, the world at large constantly refers to natural selection, adaptation, competition, and survival of the fittest as the main, if not the only, agents in natural history. What a price we pay for such backwardness! These contradictions have carried us to a dead end, particularly in the medical and social sciences, a dead end that no money and no grants can break through.

Provoked by constant criticism from inside and outside his camp, Darwin took refuge in Newton: "Newton showed how gravity manifests itself; he did not try to explain what gravity is. . . ." And he, Darwin, was not willing to go beyond the mechanism of natural selection to the variations through which it operates.

This comparison, drawn by Darwin himself, between the theory of evolution and Newtonian gravity, is of great value to us. Darwin felt that evolution is as inexplicable as gravity, that it proceeds by unknown ways. It is always and everywhere present—in prison, behind bars, subterraneously—an apple will always fall down; and the living cell, always and everywhere, tends to reproduce itself (often in a slightly improved version). A collapse of this tendency toward self-reproduction (and self-improvement) is just as unlikely and improbable as the collapse of gravitation.

IV

The mystery of the evolution of species can perhaps be clarified through the study of the development of the separate individuals. The question is how the growth of an individual, animal or plant, results in the creation of a perfect body with certain precise forms, and not in an indefinite, amorphous mass. What *directs* it, what pushes it on in one plane and limits in another?

Every part of a living creature is in harmony with other parts and with the entity. The development of an animal or plant is organized and proceeds "as toward an aim." If interference with the normal progress of an organism occurs, especially if it happens at an early stage, the living creature shows a strong tendency to regenerate the disrupted parts; it is still directed toward its "aim" which is the perfect, adult, mature specimen, capable of self-reproduction.

This development, we are told, is predetermined by the genetic units present in every cell. But how are we to understand that the actions of these units are coordinated in such manner— slowing down the growth in some parts, accelerating it in others, rhythmically expanding and organizing—that all stages in time and space are passed through without confusion or delay? Such coordination and interrelation is difficult to understand in terms of genes only, genes being *separate* units, while here something unites the entire living being, leads it, regulates and brings it to its own ideal. (Is the general endocrinic balance also conditioned by those isolated genes?)

This unity of the entire living being becomes obvious when we interfere with the normal development. The organism shows a miraculous capacity to reconstruct lost parts and to reestablish the normal course of growth, that is, to deliver the usual product by unusual roads. *The entity is present in every part.* This is the gift of self-regulation; every creature is a harmonious system, organized and perfect. It is as if the cells of an embryo were listening to a strain of music directing them in the dark; or as if every cell, besides having its own individual watch, could also refer to a Big Ben who keeps the different watches synchronized at all times. (The "aim," apparent in every creature, may also be particular to the entire body of living creatures as an entity, and to the entire organic stock.)

Wherefrom comes this capacity for organization? Well— wherefrom comes the phenomenon of gravitation? The simplest way would be to acknowledge that a supreme power (of a very complicated nature) exerts its influence uniformly throughout the cosmos, so that it is manifested as gravitation in the mineral world and as the tendency to self-reproduction or self-improvement in the organic world; consequently, confusion and pathology must result from any resistance to this universal force.

It appears certain that, throughout our history, life has been directed one way: toward more organization, complication, perfection. If a ship left port without destination and were suddenly to embark upon a definite and steady course, would it not be right to assume that there is an undercurrent carrying it in that direction, or a wind blowing, or a hidden skipper maneuvering toward a definite goal? To deny this seems madness; but this is precisely what we are doing, under the pretext of being highly scientific.

One of the most important manifestations of a living organism is the choice (perhaps the free choice on the cellular level) that it constantly has to make. The ameba already prefers some substances and rejects others it meets on its way. The higher organism rejects grafts, ejects foreign bodies, devours microorganisms, and absorbs chosen substances. When a cell stops discriminating and accepts everything (or nothing) through its membrane, we know it is dead.[39] These choices are not made capriciously, at random, but correspond to some inner ideal (present or future) of this organism. Random choices would be catastrophic in the long run, and no choice at all is equal to death. We might say that "we know where we are going but that we do not know that we know it." In that case, the entire question of culture would be to explore this inner wisdom, to move *consciously* toward this "known" goal, and to be able to reverse our course whenever necessary.

The minute, gradual changes of which Darwin spoke do not lead to mutations, which are spontaneous, distinct, and stable. The ruthless solitary leaders have less chance to leave a marked change in the progeny than the numerous little good-humored fellows around them. And this is crucial! The adrenals are large in animals that constantly have to fight or resort to flight in order to survive. The adrenals increase in size when animals are crowded into cages and subjected to fights and irritating competition.[40] Researchers have found that *adreno-cortical changes* in rats, moles, and other animals that have been crowded together appear to *check* reproduction. This explains probably the population cycles in species and nations, and shows why the South Americans and Indians reproduce so abundantly while the civilized Western executive, who is in constant competition, stops after one or two descendants.

Selye supports the theory that much of the pathology and what he calls diseases of adaptation arise from abnormally increased cortical secretion, accompanied by adrenal abnormality that is a response to stress (and may be considered a fatal result of the self-defense process).

V

Darwin's theory of natural selection could suffice to explain the origin of variations, but not the origin of species. Here the *mutations* of genes helped to save the day. It is not clear, however, why this new elaboration must be called Darwinism or neo-Darwinism.

In Mendel's experiments new species appeared suddenly (spontaneously). No intermediate steps or gradual transitions, no struggle for existence, no survival of the fittest, were required for the creation and conservation of new, stable forms. There was a distinct *gap* between the shortest specimen of a new giant mutant and the tallest specimen of the old form. And no search for the lost link seemed needed.

Mendel mated, for instance, smooth, yellow peas with wrinkled peas; in the first generation they produced only smooth yellow peas; in the next, smooth yellow, wrinkled yellow, smooth green, and wrinkled green appeared at the ratio of 6:3:3:1. The hybridization turned out to be neither equalization nor homogenization of characteristics, and the ratio of the progeny was only statistically, not individually, determined. Which parent would give a smooth yellow and which a wrinkled progeny was not predetermined (just as with the disintegration of the atom of radium). There is nothing definitive in such heredity; it is a trend, a potentiality, that can be and often is overcome. For all we know there may be freedom to choose one or the other place in the statistical order. Genetics is subject to the laws of the new microscopical physics and the principle of indetermination. Here it is worth repeating Heisenberg's statement about atoms: "They form a world of potentialities or possibilities rather than of things and facts." (This applies of course also to all our deterministic tests—I.Q., aptitude, vocational, lie detection, etc.)

"Any attempt to analyze living organisms into their simplest components must lead us to consideration of the hereditary materials, but those materials only specify the potentialities a new individual inherits from its parents."[41] Whether these potentialities necessarily become translated into reality is another question. Here the laws of probability enter into the picture and warp it, for probability has no meaning whatsoever in the *individual* case.

It is possible that all beings are not completely finished creatures: Only potencies were originally created, able to unfold themselves along certain lines. Thomas Aquinas puts it this way: "He works even to this day in the work of propagation." And Bergson: "The ape that had sufficient energy and talent to become a man was already a man." Also Richard the Englishman: "Nothing can be produced from a thing that is not contained in it." But this does not mean that everything it contains must automatically be projected.

If particles, molecules, cells, have a certain inclination and preference; if they are directed toward a definite goal and manifest a positive tendency toward self-reproduction and self-improvement, then the order of probabilities acquires a completely different aspect. When the dice are loaded (have "preferences"), one cannot naively apply general laws of probabilities and get a correct end result.

If genes are only potentialities, and if the choice takes place in a direction of preference (on the cellular level), the heredity dictum changes its character. What is true for atoms must be even more so for DNA. According to Schroedinger, "Quantum mechanics is the first theoretical aspect which accounts from first principles for all kinds of aggregates of atoms actually encountered in Nature. Consequently, we may safely assert that there is no alternative to the molecular explanation of the hereditary substance."[42]

In the wake of works by Delbruck, Schroedinger has pointed out the close analogy between the fundamental laws of genetics and the quantum theory. It appears that the immense stability of the hereditary substance corresponds to a giant molecule in a stationary state, and the mutations would then correspond to quantum jumps or isomeric forms.

The new ideas in quantum mechanics must enter the picture of biology and sociology as long as we study them on the nuclear level. Consequently, the great concepts of indetermination and complementarity should influence this entire field. Heredity is not an automatic process. It is only a question of chances and probability. And probability has no meaning in the *particular* case; it is only statistically valid. In addition, probability holds true only "if the dice are not loaded," that is, if the cells have no definite sympathy and *direction*.

To tell a couple with an abnormal gene that their child has n percent chances of being a cripple is a crime and / or madness.

VI

"It is remarkable that a science which began with the consideration of games of chance should have become the most important object of human knowledge."[43]

Let's take this case as an example of a probability with definite measure: the probability is 1/6 that the first throw of the dice will be an ace. We throw the dice, and the ace may turn up or not. Yet our conviction remains the same: the probability is still 1/6. This means that if we threw the dice 60,000 times, the ace would show about 10,000 times. Thus, though the statement refers to a *singular* throw, its meaning is not at all connected with that particular throw. This is the most striking trait of probability, so often ignored, especially by the proponents of common sense.

How would the above affect medical science whose great and only concern is the concrete *individual* case? Since the ideal of medicine is the individual case, it should not be concerned at all with "probabilities"; nevertheless, suddenly, it finds itself involved almost exclusively with masses, classes, divisions, types, categories. Statistics is the negation of the medical ideal. Stalin, a very cruel but intelligent man, sized up the situation correctly when he stated: "The death of one man is a tragedy, the death of a million is statistics."

We also have to bear in mind that probability can be evaluated only on the basis of information. This creates many complications, since the information supplied is never complete and often, at least partially, incorrect. Will it rain next April 14? What should we take into account: the frequency of rain on April 14 for the last several years; the frequency of rain on this date in years with meteorological conditions similar to the prevailing ones; a combination taking into account both conditions? Or is there still something else—e.g., the moon: full or eclipsed? Should we, in the statistics of cancer of the breast, take the pathology as an entity regardless of the extent involved? Should we separate the patients into classes and types, according to age, sexual activity, ideology, temperament, and countless other features that could have a decisive effect on the statistical picture?

What's more, we have to commit ourselves to a definite general assumption *before* we begin to compute. We cannot compute the probable position of a planet on the basis that Einstein's theory has a probability of 75 percent and Newton's a probability of 25 percent. The computer must first *commit* himself to one theory to get results of some scientific usefulness (he must do it, although he does not believe 100 percent in either theory). We may doubt information that is vouched us, but the moment we start computing, our doubts must be deferred and erased. This concerns even the question whether the dice are loaded or not. Skeptics, we must yet behave like believers—and that creates an ambiguous situation in science.

Probability is always relative to the information supplied. If false information is supplied the probability will be false; if incomplete information—the result will be incomplete, unconvincing. Now what right do we have to claim that our information in genetics and medicine is complete? Yet the results stemming from this sort of information are indiscriminately applied by our authorities, thus influencing our schools, social services and even the intimate family life. Statistics, like mathematics, is an intellectual game, often irrational, and only sometimes useful.

Logic is a poor guide in matters of nature. It is not common sense but rather uncommon sense that helps us in most problems of modern life. More difficult even to digest is the combination of common and uncommon sense, their interrelation, the free passage from rational to irrational methods, the mixing of them according to our needs. The very definition of what is and what is not rational is done rather capriciously. There seem to be no clear criteria. Absurdity still seems incompatible with good methods of thinking, although nature is full of manifestations that, though seemingly absurd, have to be acknowledged as reality. Absurdity is part of our life—not only in the theatre and great fiction; as far as science is concerned, absurdity makes definite sense.

A constant of the Absurd can be deducted by means of mathematical probability. Let's take an unwound watch and note the time at which it stopped. Obviously, even though the watch does not work and its hands do not move, it will show the correct time twice every twenty-four hours. Two times out of twenty-four, absurdity is victorious and does make sense. In other words, in $8\frac{1}{3}$ percent the watch is right. Thus we arrive at the Absurdity Constant specific for our system. It means that any procedure, any technique, any treatment, any drug, any surgery, any tool, any theory as absurd as an unwound watch, would in $8\frac{1}{3}$ cases out of a hundred give a sufficiently positive, reasonable, beneficial result. Whether we perform a radical mastectomy, a simple, or none at all, in $8\frac{1}{3}$ percent of the cases the result will be a five-year survival. Therefore a deduction of $8\frac{1}{3}$ percent should perhaps be made in all our statistical calculations, so as to evaluate correctly the actual merits of the applied process. This Absurdity Constant of ours can be readily transformed into a universal constant.

VII

The old problem of the justification of God, the theodicy, is still with us—especially among the younger, more sensitive generation. The argument goes like this: If God is the Creator of the world he is responsible for it and for all the cruelties arising in the natural order. And yet he is omnibenevolent as well as omnipotent! Needless to say that the very way the question is put is a prenuclear way of reasoning, for it implies that every effect in the universe is the consequence of a cause. Classical theology solves this critical antinomy through the concept of original sin and the fall of free man. However, youth has always felt reluctant to accept this traditional answer. Now this knot can perhaps be disentangled for them in the light of modern quantum mechanics and Bohr's complementarity principle. Matter is particle and matter is wave. God is love and God is omnipotent . . . but these two natures should be considered *complementarily* only, not simultaneously.

When we use the term "simultaneously" we do not say much. Time acquires a completely different character on the microscopic (and probably also on the supercosmic) level—if it exists there at all. The normal decay process of nucleons is of the order of 10^{-24} seconds (or less); the electron and proton have effective diameters of the order of 10^{-13} cm. The first is a fraction of a second: one divided by one with 24 zeros; the latter is a fraction of a centimeter: one divided by one with 13 zeroes. Can we apply our meaning of time to such an order of dimensions? Can immeasurable spaces and millions of light years be projected onto a three-dimensional (or even four-dimensional) concept? Immeasurable sub- and supercosmoses have something more than our measurable dimensions; they manifest contradictions: they can be this and that and still something else. We must admit and absorb this truth, once and for all, at least for arguments on the subatomic and supercosmic scale. What is matter? Wave or particle? Or neither wave nor particle and still something else? What is the Trinity? United and not One; not One and yet not separated. Does God exist? The answer may be yes and no, or not yes and not no (and still Something else). Such projections of post-quantum reasoning into humanitarian and religious fields is one of the aims of this book.

"Here is wisdom. Let him that hath understanding count the number of the beast: for it is the number of a man; and his number is Six hundred three score and six" (Rev. 13, 18). That we dare—in a book dedicated to medicine, philosophy, and modern science—that we dare seriously to quote from Saint

John is a fact of great significance. Things have changed.

Says P. A. M. Dirac: "There are some fundamental constants in nature: the charge on the electron (designated e), Planck's constant divided by 2 pi (designated h) and the velocity of light (c). From these fundamental constants one can construct a number that has no dimensions: the number hc/e^2. That number is found by experiment to have the value 137, or something very close to 137. Now, there is no known reason why it should have this value rather than some other number. Various people have put forward ideas about it, but there is no accepted theory. Still, one can be fairly sure that some day physicists will solve the problem and explain why the number has this value. There will be a physics in the future that works when hc/e^2 has the value 137 and that will not work when it has any other value.[45]

True, there is a difference between the two statements above—but there also is a definite similarity, a similarity that is of great import to us. (And incidentally, by reducing 666 to its prime factors we arrive at 37.)

Einstein describes a celestial body so voluminous that no ray of light would emerge from it due to its tremendous gravitational attraction—perhaps that same light Saint John of the Cross saw striking out from a dark cloud.

"*Credo quia absurdum.* ..." I believe because it is absurd to believe, said Tertullian. The full text is seldom quoted: "Et mortuus est Dei Filius, prorsus credibile est, quia impossibile est. Et sepultus et surrexit, certum est, quia impossibile est." The Son of God died; this can be believed since it is inconceivable. And he was buried and he resurrected; this is true because it is impossible.

Compare this with Niels Bohr's: "How wonderful that we have met with a paradox. Now we have some hope of making progress!" and with his words to Wolfgang Pauli: "We all agree that your theory is crazy. The question which separates us is whether it is sufficiently crazy to have a chance to be correct. My feeling is that it is not." (What a long way from the 19th century and Thomas Huxley's naive statement: "Science is simply common sense at its best—that is, rigidly accurate observation and merciless to fallacy and logic.")

The probability concept, too, suddenly meets the requirements of the Scriptures. "And I heard the number of them which were sealed and there were sealed a hundred and forty and four thousand . . ." (Rev. 7, 4). And further: "And whosoever was not found written in the book of life was cast into the lake of fire" (20, 15).

It appears now that all this is only a statistical determination. Modern quantum physics provides us with a new tool with which to explore religion and art as well as medicine and natural sciences, shedding new light and leading us out of certain dead ends. Some will survive five years and more after operation for cancer, others will perish. But who belongs to the first hundred and forty and four thousand is undetermined by causal factors. It is a question of personal choice and grace.

The question of grace, so obscured by the difficult experience of Saint Augustine, assumes a much simpler aspect due to quantum mechanics. The life of atoms, molecules, and cells is only statistically predetermined; individually they are free to choose. An atom of radium has—by grace—a life span of up to 10,000 years; but which atom will perish within the next second and which will go on for a millenium is up to the individual, on the nuclear level.

Is man free to choose between voluptuousness and chastity in the presence of a nude beauty? Of course he is free; though, among one hundred, n percent will give in. Grace, too, is only statistically predestined. One hundred and forty and four thousand will be saved, but which of them is up to the choice of the person.

"I want to do good, and do evil which I do not want to do," says Saint Paul. This essentially is the fight against irreversible processes. The urge toward reversibility is overpowering in all religions, especially in Christianity where redemption is the final reversal. "Today you will be with me in my Kingdom," Christ says to the robber on the cross. A thief . . . today . . . immediately . . . in Paradise—this is the complete negation of the natural order. Your garments may be soiled, bloodstained—but "whiter than snow" will they be washed, says Isaiah. What else is such a procedure but reversibility? You must be "reborn"—this too is reversibility. The liturgy is the process of resurrection; the rites are a return to a previous state of holiness and sanctity.

In economics, a post-quantum elaboration was introduced long ago and brought us out of the depression. We have in mind the theory of Lord Keynes.[46] The classic concept of free enterprise held that, unless the customer made money enabling him to pay for goods, those goods would not be delivered to him and, consequently, not be produced. Factories closed, manufactures froze, a deadly economic crisis ensued with everybody and everything standing idle.

Lord Keynes's simple idea consisted in putting the effect ahead of the cause. "What if we gave the consumer some extra money?" went the reasoning. "Would he not begin to buy necessities and commodities? The factories would start moving again, the buyer would get his job back, earn a salary, buy appliances. . . ."

This interchange of cause and effect, typical for our post-quantum era, performed an economic miracle. In even more concrete terms such reasoning could lead to the following: At the end of fifty active years a citizen will have earned a minimum of, say, $100,000, i.e., $2,000 per year. Let us advance him half of this sum on the day of his birth and thus give him a good start. He'll be able to pay it off—with large interest even.

The same trend might perhaps be established in foreign policy. The best thing that happened to the democratic countries was the victory of communism in China. If China were still under Chiang Kai-Shek or similar lords, it would have a tremendous, very dynamic, radical opposition; the entire Marxist movement on all five continents would still be under the command of Soviet Russia, which—without an ideological challenger and stuffed with nuclear warheads—would develop into the sole unchecked menace to everything outside her political orbit. Our world would simply be divided into two gigantic opposing camps, engaged in a geometrically increasing arms race. The final stage would be clear and inevitable. As it is, we see the colossal Chinese challenger more dangerous today to the Russian empire than to the Western commonwealths. We can choose our ally, and the Russians will readily fight with us against communist China. Is it not an achievement? No, not completely. For something more can be done along these lines. Why fight 800 million Chinese, even if there is a chance to win?

Could we not maneuver in such a way that China too would unite with us against another, formidable, new challenger? Indeed if some day we meet with a strange dangerous species or element in outer space threatening our way of life on earth, all this will become an immediate reality: We will suddenly become brothers to the Chinese, brothers in arms against a more dangerous enemy.

Here again, by putting the cart before the horse, by negating the cause-and-effect dictum, we could save a lot of lives (and not only Chinese lives). Such reasonings, and explorations along similar lines, are within the context of the modern post-quantum revolution and can easily be projected into the domain of religion also. Indeed, many contemporary philosophers claim that if a society worshipped a God who is Love, and acted accordingly, then, for all existential purposes, such a God would manifest himself in that society.

VIII

The new quantum mechanics also affects the domain of art and literature. It is a fact that the so-called psychological novel is becoming obsolete. Based on the cause-and-effect dictum, it reigned over Western literature for the last hundred years or more. In this sort of novel, all developments are subject to a chain of psychological events, where each link is the result of the preceding and the origin of the next: Because she said this, he did that . . . because he smiled, she went to bed. . . . This psychological determinism shows even in writers who, like Dostoevsky, knew that the nature of life and man is irrational. Such writers have to *justify* any of their spontaneous jumps from one orbit to another.

Tolstoi's *War and Peace* parallels in many ways Newton's *Principles*. The big celestial bodies still work according to the philosophy of the 18th century. Tolstoi relies directly on Laplace in his philosophy of history. Indeed—a supernatural brain could know where all the innumerable particles of the universe are, and where they are going; but no human being can calculate that—

certainly not Napoleon. A nation, like a beehive, knows unconsciously what to do in a crisis and cannot be distracted from its
salutary actions. It is because the events are predetermined that
the hero cannot sway them; if he tries to, the hero acts like a child
inside a closed carriage who imagines that he is driving the
horses.

"Just as in astronomy the difficulty of admitting the motion
of the earth lay in the immediate sensation of the earth's station-
ariness and of the planet's motion, so in history the difficulty of
recognizing the subjection of the personality to the laws of space
and time and causation lies in the difficulty of surmounting the
direct sensation of the independence of one's personality. But
just as in astronomy, the new view said, 'It is true, we do not feel
the movement of the earth, but, if we admit its immobility, we
are reduced to absurdity, while admitting its movement, we are
led to laws,' so in history, the new view says, 'It is true, we do
not feel our dependence, but admitting our freewill, we are led to
absurdity; admitting our dependence on the external world,
time, and cause, we are led to laws.' "[47]

Proust, too, is determinist, with his associations between
subjects from different fields. He constantly establishes indirect
associations and relies on them. "One may list in an interminable
description the objects that figured in the place described, but
truth will begin only when the writer takes too different objects,
establishes their relationship—analogous in the world of art to
the sole relationship in the world of science, the law of cause and
effect—and encloses them in the necessary rings of a beautiful
style, or even when, like life itself, comparing similar qualities in
two sensations, he makes their essential nature stand out clearly
by joining them in a metaphor, in order to remove them from the
contingencies of time, and links them together with the inde-
scribable bond of an alliance of words. . . ."[48] This is an ob-
lique, boomerang-like, great, but still "predetermined" way of
feeling and reasoning.

The direct flow of childish (obvious) associations of the
surrealists—Joyce included—is clearly determined and unfree
in its course. These great writers achieved great works—just as
Newton and Darwin did in science. The inadequacy appears
only when one goes down to the nuclear, microscopic level. The

contemporary writer who wants to fulfill his task must be aware of the impact of modern discoveries, in the same way that Tolstoi and Proust (and Dante) fed on the great scientific concepts of their time. A contemporary novel might incorporate the new concepts of quantum mechanics and be rather based on spontaneous, irrational, undetermined events.

Kafka, who seems to many completely irrational, is perhaps the beginning of such post-quantum literature. However, only his starting point is obscure or "absurd"; once the beginning is accepted, everything is run by the iron, inescapable logic of cause and effect. The hero of *The Trial* is persecuted, taken before a court, finally executed; till the end he does not know what the charges against him are. But he fights very rationally against an apparently absurd legal proceeding that, here, represents the irreversible process.

If we imagined for a moment that Kafka's protagonist entered a doctor's office for his yearly, routine checkup, and there, suddenly, was told that he has cancer, everything else that happens in *The Trial* would be rather trivial.

"Is it dangerous? Is there a cure? Why me, for heaven's sake, why me?" "Should I settle for symptomatic and supportive therapy or accept radical surgery?"

Finally he submits to surgery and dies on the operating table. What's enigmatic or absurd about the case?

Earlier, Tolstoi used this comparison of a patient and an accused in the *Death of Ivan Ilytch* (who *is* a judge). "It was exactly as in his court of justice. Exactly the same air as he put on in dealing with a man brought up for judgment, the doctor put on for him." And later, "The judge is coming! . . . The Judge is coming, the Judge is coming—he repeated to himself.—Here is the Judge! But I am not to blame!—he shrieked in fury—What is it for?—"

It is clear from the journal entry of December 23, 1921, that Kafka knew the *Death of Ivan Ilytch* very well and liked it best, together with the story *The Three Old Men*, amongst all of Tolstoi's works. (Franz Kafka, *Journal*, Grasset, Paris, 1954.)

The main characteristic of a novel is that it proceeds in time. It is the only art form where time is not incidental: It is made by time, devised and incarnated due to time. The novel is also the art form that did not exist before the advent of Christ. Such as we know it, the novel appeared only in our era. This is important—for time took on its concrete and real meaning only in our Judeo-Christian culture. The fact that Christ was crucified at a definite time (under Pontius Pilate) is of the same value to our theology as the fact of the incarnation per se. The ancient Greeks and Egyptians had no sense of time, no use for it, no concept of it. *Undated* Greek monuments can still be found, with inscriptions to the effect that peace was concluded here with a certain enemy "for one hundred years." A month or a year later they could consider these hundred years elapsed. The closest term for a period of time for the Greek was "era"—and that is a lot of time.

The connection of the novel with the concept of time makes it an important and perhaps unique form of Christian art. This is why the change in our concept of time must have a direct impact on the novel and must be reflected by it.

In fact there always was a miraculous tendency toward spontaneity and the absurd.

Dostoevsky had his Idiot; Tolstoi had Platon Karatayev and many simpletons who spontaneously reflected un-causal truths in what is basically a "post-quantum" intuition.

Already in antiquity the circus clown expressed reality through the absurd, and the absurd in reality. Don Quixote's madness seems complete; yet, at times, Sancho Panza appears still more irrational. Through these two exponents, Cervantes arrives at describing his reality. Captain Ahab is certainly mad; yet he is the only one who knows where he is going and why.

All these great masters of the "Newtonian" area already felt the need for the post-quantum *uncommon* sense, the need to describe the "evidence of things not seen."

Heisenberg's indetermination principle can easily be projected into the field of the arts.

If the artist describing an object, a situation, a face, makes it too beautiful, too subjective, too poetical, he distorts its reality; if he does it too slavishly, too mirrorlike, too "honestly," its inherent beauty will be lost. Thus there is always a limit (Planck's h) beyond which an artist cannot go in his creation ($dP \cdot dQ = H$).

In painting and sculpture no concept of time is involved.

Realistic painting (and not only the Soviet brand), which claims objectivity, is obsolete in the post-quantum era.

Plato envisaged the world of forms: the ideal Form of a shoe, let's say; then the world of objects, i.e., the shoe made by a shoemaker; then the world of art, a painting of this shoe by Van Gogh (or a sculpture by Rodin). The last category was the least useful and least precious in Plato's hierarchy. What Plato saw was either a shoe—or not a shoe. The concept of complementarity escaped him totally.

But the impressionists saw it: It is a house and, yet, not a house; it is something else and perhaps not something else. Their interest in color and light was undoubtedly influenced by experiments in the physics of color carried out by Chevreul (1786–1889). The new idea was that an object of any given color casts a shadow tinged with its *complementary*: thus a great movement in painting started.

Says Picasso: "The big thing in modern painting is this. A painter like Tintoretto, for example, starts on his canvas, and then he continues, and when he finally has covered it and worked it all over, only then is the canvas completed. While if you take a painting by Cézanne (and this is even more obvious in his water colors), the moment he puts the first stroke of the brush the painting is already there."

Of course, if we go back in history, we can find great souls who already in the Middle Ages painted in accordance with a "quantum mechanics" concept. Surely some philosophers, saints, and scientists had a precognition of it, too. And the teaching of the great churches was always on this post-nuclear level. (The Body and Blood are not separated in the bread and wine but both are in both!)

All sciences should rely more and more on this irrational, spontaneous interpenetration peculiar to art and religion, where disengagement and reengagement between object and subject takes place constantly. And art (if not religion) should get acquainted with the quantum state of matter—if we are in earnest about wanting to acquire a full knowledge of existing reality. For this purpose a new mentality and a new semantics must be established; (in this respect, we can and must learn a great deal from the East.)

"The veil" still covers tightly the secrets of nature; violence, disease, and death are the consequence of this riddle, this enigma, this seal. The discovery of reality, of the truth, is an aspect of the general fight for control and reversibility. Irreversible processes have haunted mankind from antiquity; many of them have been reversed, many more can still be reversed.

This consistent trend toward reversibility in our Western culture cannot be a simple coincidence. It must be the expression of a fundamental need and knowledge.

The American Constitution claims that all men are created equal. This is not true. From the "natural" point of view men are not created equal. It is our will and our choice that can reverse that natural order and *make* us equal, not only legally but biologically and spiritually as well.

IX

There is an inner call to "reverse" our course by seeking the lost paradise, and also by denying a "natural" order of which death and irreparability are the crowning end. Psychiatry has tried to establish the most potent mainspring of man. For Freud it was sex; for Adler, power, ambition. How much more real is the tendency toward reversibility!

We reverse the natural order not only by fighting disease and restoring youth. Every time we answer an offense with a smile or a good word, or do not return a stroke (and what could be more unnatural!), we reverse the natural course of events, break the chain of cause and effect, and establish a new, free, undeterministic order. Whenever the omnibenevolent God is worshipped, the deterministic laws of Darwin, Marx, Pavlov, Freud, et al., are reversed. Such worship can spring only from the inner urge of the person toward reversibility or from a horror of irreversibility.

For those concerned with the process of reversibility the direction of time is even more important than the very concept of time. "On the subatomic scale there may be no consistent direction of time and so time as we normally understand it may be essentially a macroscopic phenomenon."[49] We would rather say:

Time is *only* a macroscopic phenomenon, meaning that on the supra-cosmic scale it is also completely different.

The concept of the reversibility of time demands some explanations. It is in no way a negation of time and a change of the meaning of life. Reversibility of time does not imply a complete turn in the opposite direction. If *all* processes in the universe were reversed, we should have precognition instead of memory. And there would be nothing special in this situation: Everything would become symmetrically reversed and would seem exactly as it is now.[50]

Actually, this would present a *double* reversal: of all the events, and of our sense of past-present-future. This double reversal, like a negation of the negative, would leave everything unchanged. The *recoverability* of an original situation is the main thing, not the numerical reversal of steps and stages. Reversibility is restorability.[51]

When we speak about a dynamic reversibility, we assume that all events of which we are already aware will still be assigned to the past, and the work accomplished (created) by us will *not* retract or vanish. If we play a sonata backwards, we still recognize a tune and can distinguish it from other tunes. A major scale, played forward or backward, remains a major scale.

Reversibility of time is not an annihilation of our history. On the contrary, it is because our past *is* so important to us that we have the urge to approach it again some day and correct it in the light of our new experience. In a universe where time is reversed, entropy and disorder decrease.

The great whale accomplished a reversal and went back into the ocean. But this did not wipe out the fact that he had become a mammal and had lived on the earth.

Here is one image of reversibility in our terms.

X

The established order, which in its causal chain from birth to death seems irreversible, is a formidable challenge. The common man, who is usually not able to fight this "natural" order creatively, takes to drink or breaks windows as a way of protest and of confirming his own person in this elusive world.

Tolstoi put it clearly in *War and Peace*: "It was the same feeling that impels the volunteer-recruit to drink up his last farthing, the drunken man to smash looking-glasses and window-panes for no apparent cause, though he knows it will cost him his little all; the feeling through which a man in doing things, vulgarly speaking, senseless, as it were, proves his personal force and power, by manifesting the presence of a higher standard of judging life, outside mere human limitations."

Indeed, we have no way in our modern life to express this tendency but by acts that are often, by their very nature, against the law. Under our civilization, those acts through which the individual can break away from the vicious chain of cause and effect must, by definition, more often than not be senseless and void. Murder, rape, suicide, head the list of our "free" choices against the established order.

The existentialists know the great meaning of the act; the trouble is that they cannot find a way to act. Sartre's heroes filch books from the stands on the Boul' Mich' or chase after minors, when they want to act.

The so-called juvenile delinquents, at a loss how to assert themselves in the confusing stream of life, unite in gangs, smoke marijuana, engage in crime; but here, too, the basis is that same tendency not to accept the irreversible, a tendency that could be converted and put to good use.

The "hippies" dress in medieval costumes, walk around barefoot, wear garments of leather or skin—in a frank attempt to live another life, to have a second chance by reversing into a different epoch and thus escape or postpone the bleak future. All this is an obvious manifestation of the inner quest for reversibility. The sad thing about these youths is that by indulging in hallucinatory drugs they distort reality (or the senses of perception) and thus defeat their purpose.

And yet, escapes from the cause-and-effect dictum are always within our reach, here and now. To offer the other cheek is certainly a reversal of our entire system. In our jungles full of fossilized prophets, such as Adam Smith, Malthus, Darwin, Newton, and Marx, it demands a truly heroic effort to stop the ugly chain of reactions. The individual is not prepared for such a *tour de force*; our civilization conditions us for exactly the opposite. We may possess some other, deeper, knowledge on the cellular, molecular, nuclear level, but on the level of organs and organisms, consciously, we are directed toward merciless fight and self-defense (which is suicide).

A new trend could be established in our society, a trend more akin to the modern laws of physics and biology which reflect a spiritual reality. But first of all, the old pseudoscientific theories have to be officially given up in medicine and the social sciences, just as they have been abolished in modern physics.

CONCLUSIONS

Having come to the end, I still feel the need to sort out some of the issues.

In the first parts I described the misery of contemporary medicine despite the miraculous progress in research, skill, and technique. The experiments are great, the doctors are capable and good, funds are available, but the entire discipline is lagging far behind other branches of science. This misery of modern medicine is due to the inadequacy of its philosophy, a philosophy still based on 18th century concepts.

In order to prove this point I reviewed the essential features of modern science and demonstrated that modern science has long since changed, revised, or abandoned what is still considered "scientific" and up-to-date in medicine and the social sciences.

The recent revolution in physics had no repercussions in the social sciences and in medicine. The concept of gravitation, in a new space-time continuum, has changed significantly. The laws of thermodynamics are no longer completely valid; entropy with its heat death is not necessarily true; global reversibility is the order of the day; the idea of a *perpetuum mobile* comes back, rehabilitated; and the universe is no longer thought of as isolated.

The advent of the new quantum mechanics has manifested an uncommon (perhaps absurd) dual reality, dual at least in its projection; a reality of particles *and* waves (perhaps neither particles nor waves); and the indetermination principle returned spontaneity and freedom of will to nature—at least on the nuclear level. Thus we are no longer bound to the dictum of cause and effect to which our sciences have so long been chained.

Darwin's famous natural selection and survival of the fittest, which supposedly brought about the entire evolution from an ameba to the Huxleys, are no longer taken at their face value. The introduction of genetics, with the inexplicable jumps (muta-

149

tions), and a reevaluation of Lamarck do away with Darwinism. It cannot be saved by simply changing its name to neo-Darwinism.

The cell does manifest a definite tendency and direction. Genes are only potentialities and, as such, present statistical determination, not a dynamic, *individual*, cause-and-effect link. Probability, so influential in modern science, has nothing to do with the individual (next) case; the global application of this principle in medicine, law, or the social sciences, where the individual is the goal, is therefore contradictory and unscientific.

Concepts arisen from modern quantum mechanics have not been projected onto fields where they could present a powerful tool for exploring new domains. In religion, the theology of the Trinity, and a solution of the theodicy, can be supported by the irrational concept of the nature of matter as dual (and one). And—as long as the freedom of a photon or an electron has been established, the freedom of a person does not present any real problem. (Predestination, like determination, has only statistical value.)

In art, too, the disposal of the causality principle must have repercussions. First of all—a new novel can emerge, a novel not based on psychological or any other determinism.

We say that the cell manifests a *tendency* to reproduce itself (and, perhaps, in an improved form—a form previously "known" to it). This actually is a quest for reversibility. Science, art, politics, law, economics, and, of course, religion take part in this process. Culture is inversely proportional to the amount of irreversible processes still remaining in a given society.

The worst among all the mistakes supported by our old theories is the notion of the self-defense mechanism as always beneficial. This is wrong, at least for our stage of the game! If the cell has any interest in survival it must try hard to rid itself of much of this obsolete information that was automatically passed on to it by the notorious DNA.

One of the tasks of contemporary medicine is to initiate the person into possibilities for control and reeducation of his autonomous centers, to teach him how to prevent panicky, blind overstretching of the system: The patient should cease to think and talk exclusively about himself, his profit, his comfort, and handicaps. A permanent state of well-being cannot be achieved in a fragmented, disunified world.

NOTES

1. V. A. Negovsky, "Some Results of the Physiopathological Study of Terminal States." *Arch. int. Pharmacodyn.*, 1962, CXL, No. 1–2, Brussels, Belgium.

2. *Medical Tribune, May 6, 1964.*

3. Donald E. Hale, *Anesthesiology.* F. A. Davis, Philadelphia, 1955.

4. John C. McDermott, "Reflections on Hysterectomy," condensed from *California Medicine* 96:96, 1962 (CMD May, 1962).

5. Max Planck, *The New Science.* Greenwich Editions, 1959. (The Universe in the Light of Modern Physics, p. 179).

6. Max Schur, "New Light on Sigmund Freud's Thought on Death," *Medical Tribune*, weekend ed., Dec. 26–27, 1964.

7. *Medical Tribune*, "Reduction in Resistance Due to Surgery, X-ray may speed metastases," May 6, 1963.

8. Walter B. Cannon, *Bodily Changes in Pain, Hunger, Fear and Rage.* Harper Torchbooks, 1963.

9. H. Kunz, E. Domanig, Jr., and L. Howanietz, *Causes of Postoperative Death.* Langenbecks Arch. für Klinische Chirurgie, Berlin (Cond. JAMA, June 23, 1962).

10. J. Thorwald, *The Dismissal.* Pantheon, 1962.

11. New York *Daily News*, August 6, 1962, "Jury Decides When to Remove Toxin in Uremia" (Family Doctor).

12. D. Agostino, and E. E. Cliffton, *Anesthetic Effect on Pulmonary Metastases in Rats.* Arch. Surg. 88:735, May 1964.

13. René Leriche, *La Philosophie de la Chirurgie.* Flammarion, 1951 (p. 184).

14. JAMA, Nov. 24, 1962: United Kingdom—Fatigue Test for Pilots, p. 880.

15. N. Fedorov, *The Philosophy of the Common Cause.* Charbin, 1926.

16. Hubert Larcher, *Le Sang Peut-il Vaincre la Mort.* Gallimard, 1957.

17. M. Schur, "New Light on Sigmund Freud's Thoughts on Death." *Medical Tribune*, Dec. 26–27, 1964.

18. *Medical Tribune*, Nov. 13–14, 1965.

19. *Medical Tribune*, American College of Surgeons, Atlantic City, 1965.

19a. V. Vernadsky, Selected Writings, Academy of Sciences, USSR 1954–1960.

20. Sir James Jeans, *Physics and Philosophy.* University of Michigan Press.

21. A. Robb, *The Absolute Relations of Time and Space.* Cambridge, 1921.

22. H. Poincaré, *The Value of Science.* New York, 1929.

23. Max Planck, *Where is Science Going?* Greenwich Meridian (Chapter 6).

24. Marian Smoluchovski, *Pisma*, T.3, p. 68. Warsaw, as reported in *Moskva*, 1958, *Phil. voprossi sovrem. physiky.*

25. David Bohm, *Causality and Chance in Modern Physics.* Harper Torch Book, 1957.

26. Fred Hoyle, *Nature of the Universe*. Mentor Book.
27. Niels Bohr, *Atomic Theory and the Description of Nature*. Cambridge University Press.
28. Louis de Broglie, *Matter and Light*. The New Physics, Dover, N.Y.
29. Niels Bohr, *Atomic Physics and Human Knowledge*. Science Edit.
30. David Bohm, *Causality and Chance in Modern Physics*. Harper Torch Book, 1957.
31. Pierre Teilhard de Chardin, "The Phenomenon of Man," *Harper*, 1959.
32. Victor F. Weisskopf, *Knowledge and Wonder*. Doubleday Anchor Books.
33. Charles Darwin, *The Descent of Man*, 1st ed., as quoted by G. Himmelfarb, *Darwin and the Darwinian Revolution*. Doubleday, 1959, p. 347.
34. Charles Darwin, *The Descent of Man*, 1st ed., as quoted by L. S. Davitashvili, *V. O. Kovalevski*, Moscow, 1951.
35. H. Korschinsky, *Heterogenesis and Evolution*. Naturwissenschaftl. Wochenschrift, 14, 273, 1899; as reported by Philip G. Fothergill, *Historical Aspects of Organic Revolution*. Philosophical Library, New York, 1953.
36. Peter Kropotkin, *Mutual Aid: A Factor of Evolution*.
37. Marston Bates, *Where Winter Never Comes*. Scribner, 1952.
38. Marston Bates, *The Nature of Natural History*. Scribner, 1950.
39. Edmond W. Sinnott, *La Biologie de l'Esprit*. Gallimard.
40. John J. Christian, *The Endocrine Constellation*, as reported in *M.D.*, March 1965.
41. C. H. Waddington, *The Nature of Life*. Atheneum, 1962.
42. E. Schroedinger, *What is Life*. New York.
43. Laplace, *Théorie Analytique de Probabilité*.
44. Sir Arthur Eddington, *New Pathways in Science*, p. 123.
45. P. A. M. Dirac, "The Evolution of the Physicist's Picture of Nature," *Scientific American*, May 1963.
46. J. M. Keynes, *The General Theory of Employment, Interest and Money*. 1936.
47. L. Tolstoi, *War and Peace*.
48. Marcel Proust, *Time Recovered*.
49. G. Witrow, *The Natural Philosophy of Time*. Harper, 1963.
50. J. C. Smart, *Analysis*, 14, 1954.
51. P. W. Bridgman, *The Nature of Thermodynamics*, Harper.